Getting
the Sex
You Want

This book is dedicated to Bruce,
who has shown me true passion and love.

Text © 2008 Tammy Nelson

First published in the USA in 2008 by
Quiver, a member of
Quayside Publishing Group
100 Cummings Center
Suite 406-L
Beverly, MA 01915-6101
www.quiverbooks.com

12 11 10 09 08   1 2 3 4 5

ISBN-13: 978-59233-301-1
ISBN-10: 1-59233-301-X

Library of Congress Cataloging-in-Publication Data
Nelson, Tammy.
     Getting the sex you want : shed your inhibitions and reach
     new heights of passion together / Tammy Nelson.
          p.   cm.
     ISBN 1-59233-301-X
     1. Imago relationship therapy. 2. Marital psychotherapy.
     3. Communication in sex. I. Title.
     RC488.5.N45 2008
     616.89'1562--dc22
                              2007051459

Book design and layout: Rachel Fitzgibbon

Printed and bound in USA

Getting the Sex You Want

Shed Your Inhibitions and Reach New Heights of Passion Together

Tammy Nelson, L.P.C.

QUIVER

CONTENTS

INTRODUCTION

In my clinical work as a psychotherapist over the past twenty years, I have discovered that couples have a greater likelihood of staying together, and for longer periods of time, when they improve their sexual communication skills.

Unfortunately, the therapeutic world has had little training in helping couples explore their sexuality and communicate their erotic needs. If therapists are inexperienced when it comes to talking about sex, how can they help their clients work on these issues in their relationships?

Using a communication method called the "Imago dialogue," I have developed specific techniques that have helped men and women recharge their relationships, and bring passion back into their lives. It's not unusual for couples to be relieved after learning how to talk about their fantasies and fears and discovering what can happen just from doing the exercises in these chapters. Anyone who hopes to be in a satisfying relationship can benefit from this work (and play!).

Learning ways to communicate about sex can help you become a better lover; you will bring more skills to your relationship. The intensity and eroticism will deepen, and the passion between you and your partner can connect the two of you for life.

Using the Imago dialogue is a new way of exploring your sexuality together that can bring you to new places. It provides you with a structure in which to explore your deepest fantasies and desires. It will give you the safety to talk to each other and finally experience being seen and heard. You will find a new way to ask for the sex you have always wanted. Perhaps there are parts of your sex life that you currently enjoy. There might also be some new things you would like to try. Maybe you have sexual desires that you have been afraid to talk about. Now you will have a language in which to express these desires.

Imago therapy was developed by Harville Hendrix, the author of the best-selling book, *Getting the Love You Want*. His book has helped thousands of couples around the world ask for what they want and express their love for each other. Now you can use these time-tested techniques to expand your lovemaking and experience the intimacy and connection that will give you the passion you want and create a truly long-lasting partnership.

When you learn how to talk openly about sex, you will experience a greater level of intimacy and safety in your relationship. Loving feelings will then naturally increase toward your partner. A vital and healthy interest in sex along with a passionate curiosity for life are the ways to keep your relationship alive for a very long time.

Long-Term Passion Starts with Early Communication

"Imago: An idealized mental image of another person or the self."

—*The Merriam-Webster Dictionary*

"Normal wife" closes her book and lies back on her pillows, exhausted. She listens for the kids, wondering whether they will get up for water or to use the bathroom. The night before, both children had climbed into bed with her and her husband and she wonders whether they are both coming down with colds.

She remembers that she has forgotten to check the dryer and let the cat in for the night. She thinks about getting up, but her feet are cold and she snuggles down deeper into the bed. Every muscle aches from her day—running to the grocery store, cleaning out her son's closet, picking up her husband's shirts at the dry cleaners, and painting the hall bathroom. She scratches her head for a moment, running her fingers through her hair and tries to remember whether she took a shower that day. Her flannel shirt and boxer shorts are warm and she closes her eyes for just a moment.

Another thought suddenly occurs to her. She wonders whether her husband will want to have sex tonight. She rolls over and pretends to sleep.

"Average husband" sits in bed with his laptop balanced on his knees. He peruses the long list of e-mails he has still not opened from work that day. He glances over at his wife as she snuggles down lower in the bed. He sees she is wearing her flannel shirt. He wonders whether this is the signal that there will be no sex again tonight.

Sighing, he turns back to his computer and flips down through his e-mails until he comes to one unfamiliar e-mail address. Unsure whether it is spam, he hesitates for a moment, and then clicks on it. It is a poorly disguised invitation to visit a porn site. He sneaks another glance at his wife, and she rolls over onto her side away from him. He clicks on the link. His computer screen immediately flashes onto a catalog of young, busty, half-clad girls promising to fulfill all of his erotic dreams. He moves his cursor over one particular girl, who looks him in the eye, and he clicks on her image. A larger shot of her, with her legs spread open, invites him to charge $9.99 to his credit card for another peak, to go deeper into the site.

He sighs, and taking his glasses off of his face, rubs his tired eyes. What he really wants is to have sex with his wife, to feel connected to her. But he wonders where the passion and energy have gone.

Getting over the Fear of Talking about Sex

Marriage and long-term cohabitation breed familiarity, which can lead to a mundane erotic life. Marital familiarity can be comforting, but it doesn't lend itself to intense passion and sexual connection.

Learning to communicate sexual needs and desires early in a relationship can help contribute to an easier and smoother erotic connection later on. Sometimes it's scary to talk about sex, especially in the beginning phases of a relationship. And yet, an early pattern of relating to each other in an open and honest way can make sex more rewarding later on. Consider the following example:

Girlfriend "A" lies under Boyfriend "B." It is a Saturday night, and they are having sex. Missionary style.

This feels good, she thinks, but she wonders whether she should try and tell him that she would like to make love in a different way, using a new position. They have had sex in the missionary position every Saturday night for weeks now. How can she talk to him about what she would really like?

He seems to try so hard, she thinks. Her thoughts jump around as she lies under him: "I don't want to make him think I don't appreciate how hard he

He wonders whether his girlfriend will still want to have sex with him if he can't perform like the porn stars. His performance is a large part of what makes him feel like a man.

is trying to please me. But I wonder what else there is? And I wonder if he would mind if I used my own hand to give myself an orgasm? I don't think I could ever ask him that. I wonder if I should just fake an orgasm and make him feel good?"

As Boyfriend "B" pumps into his girlfriend he worries that he might lose his erection. It has never happened before, but he has heard stories from his buddies that sometimes they have a tough time staying hard. He wonders whether she will still want to have sex with him if he can't perform like the porn stars. His performance is a large part of what makes him feel like a man. What happens if he can't always please her?

"What if I can't last?" he thinks. "What if I come too soon?"

He keeps pushing inside her, trying not to focus on how good it feels. He begins to feel more anxious. He wonders whether he can hold out until she climaxes. He wonders whether he will he know when she comes.

"How long does it take her to come?" he thinks to himself.

He has never asked her, nor has she told him. He would like to know because he wants desperately to please her. He begins to feel the buildup and knows he is getting closer to ejaculating.

"Oh, boy, please let me last," he thinks. "I need to try harder not to think about what feels so good. This can't be the way it's supposed to be. Aren't I supposed to be gazing into her eyes or something? Maybe I should think about baseball."

Getting the Erotic Connection

Like the couples above, many people are not having the sex they really want and they aren't talking about it. Most couples want more sex, or better sex, and they don't know how to ask for it. How do we get the sex we really want? And how do we tell our partner what our fantasies are?

By using a technique called the Imago dialogue, this book will teach you and your partner ways to resexualize your partnership and have the erotic connection you truly desire. Exercises will teach you how to increase passion and connection with your partner. Writing exercises will help you clarify what you need in your erotic life—you will discover what your fantasies are and what your sexual needs are all about. You'll learn better ways to communicate with one another and talk about your deepest desires.

If you practice these skills, you *will* get the sex you want!

Introducing Imago

Imago relationship therapy was created by Harville Hendrix and Helen Hunt, authors of the book *Getting the Love You Want*, a national best-seller describing a revolutionary new way to love. The development of Imago relationship therapy is based on the theory that we choose a partner, many times unconsciously, who is perfectly suited to us, based on our image, or *imago* in Latin, that we have created from all of our experiences from childhood.

These partners have the unique ability to heal our childhood wounds. They have qualities that are similar to the positive and negative qualities of our original caretakers, and cleverly, we have chosen them because they hold the special characteristics that, when combined with our own personality traits, will help us to finish all of our unfinished business from childhood. We will get the love we always wanted! It is no coincidence that we choose the mates we do based on their similarities to and differences from our childhood experiences.

Because of this amazing and uncanny ability we all have to pick our partner, we end up with someone who can also bring up all of our issues! Although our partners can heal us from our pain like no one else, they can also hurt us in some of the same places where we have leftover wounds from childhood.

This is why relationships seem like such hard work sometimes—and why they feel so painful.

We continue to be wounded again and again in the same places that have hurt since we were young. Our partners have an almost magical way of poking us in those vulnerable places like no one else can. And yet we seem determined to continue our old behaviors, hoping against hope that if we keep repeating the same thing over and over, we will somehow get our partner to stop wounding us and give us the love we really want.

On the other hand, the partner we choose often fills our needs from childhood that were left out of our parenting. Even in the best of childhoods, we sometimes don't get our needs met. Mom doesn't always hear us when we cry; Dad doesn't always come running when we are hungry. And that's okay. Having "good enough" parents enables us to grow up and take care of ourselves as independent, functioning adults.

We then fall in love with people because we love who we are when we are with them. We feel they fulfill us in ways we cannot feel fulfilled alone. We feel safe, connected, and relaxed.

However, when they no longer complete us, or fulfill all of our needs, we no longer love ourselves when we are with them. We then withdraw from them or attack them. We are no longer quite sure how to get our needs met. We enter a power struggle or conflict stage. We either run away or settle in. If we decide to stay, we put on the old sweatpants and prepare for the long haul. This is the point where the sexual needs in the relationship begin to get split off. The sex slows down. The passion wanes. We no longer feel "in love." Some of us split off from our sexual needs; others compartmentalize their need for sex into a box deep inside themselves.

Sometimes we have a fantasy that if we trade in our partners for someone new, we might be happier. And sometimes we do. And for a while that new relationship feels better because we get to experience the romantic phase again, and all is well. However, slowly we slide back into conflict and out come the sweatpants, and we find ourselves back in that power struggle place where sex becomes maintenance sex and sometimes even part of the power struggle.

To avoid this scenario and to stay connected and experience romance and passion over the long term, communicating is the first step. But communicating is not the only step. Having a safe way to talk will increase the passion in your partnership, and many times that passion will improve your communication. Taking the first step toward communicating means sitting down together and starting with exercises like the one described below, exchanging appreciation the Imago way.

The Difference between Dialogue and Conversation

Often when we are talking with our partners—particularly when it's over a conflict—we don't really listen. We have a tendency to prepare our "rebuttal" before they even finish their sentence. We respond and cut them off before they say what they wanted to say. They then don't feel heard. And they don't feel seen for who they are.

Using the Imago dialogue, couples can practice really listening to each other and asking for what they need in the relationship. This way of communicating can go a long way toward healing our unmet needs. It can also bring us the love we truly want.

Participating in a conversation is different than being in a dialogue. Being in a dialogue means you are each totally present and in the moment, that is, you are focused solely on what your partner is saying, and not on what your response is going to be. When we listen intensely to what our partners are saying, we are more available to hear what they are trying to tell us. They experience us differently in those moments. They feel our presence, and not our distraction.

We can use the Imago process to reconnect sexually and improve our intimacy. The beginning steps of creating long-term, passionate partnerships involve working on the erotic connection as well as the companionship piece of our relationships. This includes learning to talk about sexual needs. The way to do this is to feel safe enough to share our desires and fantasies with our partner. Using the structure of the Imago dialogue, this sometimes difficult conversation becomes an experience of being deeply held and listened to by our partner.

Participating in a conversation
is different than being in a dialogue. Being
in a dialogue means you are focused solely on
what your partner is saying, and not on what
your response is going to be.

Beginning the Imago Dialogue

The Imago dialogue process involves two people—the person doing the talking—the **sender**—and the other person who is listening—the **receiver**.

For our partners to hear us, or "receive" the information we want to "send" them, we have to somehow pave the way. In other words, we have to make it safe. Most of us get defensive right away when our partners are trying to have a "serious" conversation with us. We are afraid of being criticized or that we will have to defend ourselves from something we may have done wrong. We also want to make sure they are able to hear what we are saying.

The best way to create safety for them is to start off all of our dialogues with an **appreciation.** Most of us respond well when we hear positive feedback about ourselves. So, we always start a dialogue with something we appreciate about our partner. An appreciation is something that we like about our partner. Perhaps it is an action that he has taken, or something he has done that has meaning for you. Perhaps it is a part of her personality that you love.

For instance, telling your partner that you appreciate him can mean recognizing something he does. Perhaps you normally wouldn't take the time to mention it. These can be simple things, such as "How nice he remembered that I like my coffee with sugar instead of cream." Or "I really appreciate that she came to therapy with me." Or "I am so appreciative that he mowed the lawn."

Appreciations are a way of getting more of what we want, and also a way of softening our relationship with our partner. Often our partners do things in our daily life that we appreciate but neglect to mention, when a few words from us could mean so much to them. Our relationship becomes softer when there is less tension and criticism and more positive feedback.

Try this exercise with your partner. Remember there is no right or wrong way to do this. This is the beginning of practicing a new way of talking and relating to your partner. It may feel awkward at first. That's fine. Try it anyway! Fumbling around is one way we learn how to do something that we haven't mastered yet.

EXERCISE
Exchanging Appreciations the Imago Way

For this first exercise, you will need at least fifteen minutes of uninterrupted private time together. Find a quiet place where you can sit comfortably facing each other in chairs, on the floor, or on a bed, and maintain eye contact for the entire exercise.

You are beginning the process of a new form of communication, the Imago dialogue. You will build on this format throughout the book, creating a safe structure to talk about your relationship, and later your erotic needs and fantasies. Let's start by sharing some appreciations, and learning how to **mirror** each other. This is a basic dialogue skill, explained below, and one we will use for many of the more advanced exercises to come.

This exercise will feel awkward and even a little corny in the beginning. The words may feel stilted and forced at first. Don't worry about that yet. Let the exercise feel awkward for now. Later it will feel more comfortable and you will use the technique effortlessly while talking about more erotic topics.

You may find yourself giggling or breaking eye contact. That's fine. You may feel the urge to get up and look in the refrigerator or make a phone call or check your e-mail. Try to stay focused on the exercise for the duration of both sending and receiving. The sender is the first one to talk, and the receiver is the first one to listen.

Step One
First, choose who will be the sender and who will be the receiver. The sender will talk, and the receiver's only job is to listen and mirror exactly what the sender says. **Mirroring means saying back what the sender has said with no other comments.**

Step Two

Senders will say or "send" over three things they appreciate about their partner. An example might be the following:

Sender: "I appreciate that you are having a dialogue with me tonight."

Step Three

After each appreciation, receivers will simply repeat, or mirror, what the sender has said. Continuing the example above, the receiver will simply say back while maintaining eye contact, "You appreciate that I am having a dialogue with you tonight."

In all Imago dialogues, there are only two responses a receiver might have:

1. "Please send that again" if they didn't understand or remember what they heard. Then the sender would simply repeat it and the receiver would try mirroring again.

2. Receivers mirror back what the sender says and then ask, "Is there more?"

The sender can say "yes" and send more or "no" and stop there. After three appreciations, the sender switches and becomes the receiver.

Exploring Sexual Curiosity with Empathy

The possibility of waking up a partnership and experiencing that erotic charge again sometimes feels impossible. And yet, throughout our life cycle, we continue to have erotic needs and crave intimacy through sex.

The way to increasing the erotic connection in a relationship is to begin talking to each other and empathizing with your partner. Mirroring is the first step in using these exercises, where you will practice sharing and listening.

You will, through this book, come to understand normal erotic curiosity. Erotic curiosity is simply a way to define our thoughts, fantasies, and sexual desires. We all have curiosity about things that are sexual, and we explore erotic thoughts and fantasies in our minds all the time, even if we don't

(continued on page 18)

Exploring Sexual Curiosity (continued)

share these thoughts with our partner. Understanding our partners' erotic fantasy life will help us understand what will make them happy and give us clues about what will give them a passionate, loving partnership.

In our relationship, sexual empathy needs to be present to make exploring fantasies safe. Sexual empathy means feeling connected to your partner so that you can share your fantasies. If you know that you will not be judged or dismissed by your lover for having erotic curiosity, then you will be more likely to share those thoughts.

Sexual empathy does not mean your partner will agree with your thoughts and fantasies or want to act them out with you. Sexual empathy instead means that you understand that these are your partner's erotic thoughts, and not your own. Empathy also includes being happy that your partner feels safe enough to share them with you. Feeling safe enough in a relationship to share your fantasies is a big step toward finding passion and connection.

However, we can only share our fantasies when we feel safe and respected. If we know that our partner will listen and mirror back what we are saying without judgment, then we will be more likely to share our thoughts and desires.

The Imago dialogue process is a great way to make this happen. If we can share our erotic thoughts and fantasies in a dialogue, our partner simply mirrors back what we are saying and doesn't have to respond. We then feel listened to and heard. We can talk without fear that there will be any response at all, either positive or negative. This creates a space for the fantasy to be expressed.

Sexual empathy means your partner will listen to your erotic thoughts and hold that space. We will talk more about how to be a more sexually empathetic partner later on in this book.

18   GETTING THE SEX YOU WANT

The Risk of Revealing Yourself

Talking about sex can be hard, even with a partner you have known for years. We think that the longer we are in a relationship with a partner, the easier it will be to communicate what we really want in bed. It's not. It actually becomes more difficult, because in the beginning of a relationship there is less to lose.

We take different risks in our sexuality. In the beginning of a relationship, we are able to share parts of ourselves in ways that we later repress. As we begin to feel safe with our partner, our sex becomes "safer," and we shut down the more wild parts of us for fear of hurting our partner or hurting the safety of our connection. If our relationship is to remain safe, we strive to keep the sex safe.

One of the ways that couples can begin to share their fantasies is through this next exercise, in which we will build and expand upon the first exercise. Using the appreciation dialogue outlined above, we will add to what we've learned, creating a safe space to begin to talk about sex. This is a great way for couples to create an opening in which an erotic conversation can happen. Remember, appreciation is the way to create that opening. If you want to get your needs met, appreciation is the doorway in.

EXERCISE
Starting to Talk about Sex

For this exercise, you will need at least twenty-five minutes of uninterrupted private time together. Find a quiet place where you can sit comfortably facing each other in chairs, on the floor, or on a bed to maintain eye contact for the entire exercise.

You may want to turn down the lights, put on soft music, light some candles, and put on comfortable and sexy clothes. Setting the right mood is a great way to get started, and can help lead to more passion later on.

First, we'll start by again sharing appreciations and mirroring each other. This is a basic dialogue skill, and one we will use for many of the more advanced exercises to come. This may still feel awkward, but you may have now felt some of the nice feelings that come with the experience of being mirrored. The words may still feel

(continued on page 20)

(continued)

stilted and forced. Don't worry. How fast you get this is not a reflection of how much you care about each other. Let the exercise feel awkward for now. Giggle, squirm, blush, and feel silly… it's all normal.

Try to stay focused on the exercise for the duration of both sending and receiving.

Step One

First, choose who will be the sender and who will be the receiver. Senders will "send" over one thing they appreciate about their partner. Receivers will mirror back what the sender says.

Step Two

Senders will send over one thing they appreciate about their partner sexually. Receivers will mirror this back as well.

Step Three

Finally, senders will say one thing they really like sexually and would like more of. Receivers should try not to comment on what their partner is saying, but just mirror back exactly. This is important. The receiver does not need to agree, make promises, refuse, make excuses, or answer in any way. There does not need to be any response whatsoever. This exercise is only about mirroring.

Again, there are only two responses a receiver might make—"please send that again," or the receiver can mirror back what the sender says and then ask, "Is there more?" The sender then can say "yes" and send more or "no" and stop there.

Now that you have shared your appreciations for each other, how do you feel? Can you tell your partner what it was like to hear those things? Try not to judge what you heard, or disagree, or argue. You do not have to agree, compromise, or commit. Just sit with what you heard. You can ask questions, but try to soak up the appreciation for now.

The History of Love

Men and women have different emotional needs, and physically respond differently during sex. But we have one thing in common—we are all looking for love.

"Eros," or the creative urge to love, is also the drive to stay alive and to live passionately. Eros is what makes us feel desire in our relationships, giving us that wonderful, energized feeling that we all long for. This is the energy we call passion.

Love is natural; it is the instinct for passion, or the Eros urge. Eros was a figure from Greek mythology; the son of Aphrodite, the Greek goddess of love. As the representation of all that was passionate, romantic, and sexual, Eros was worshipped as a god of fertility—he was the *life* urge. Ancient Greeks felt Eros represented unbridled sexual passion. Yet he was also famous, like Cupid, for being deceitful, overly playful, and unfaithful to his lovers. In English, "Eros" is the root of the word *erotic*.

The Romans had their own interpretation of Eros; they called him Cupid, the god of love. Cupid tortured his lovers with arrows that put them under his spell and left them powerless. The name *Cupid* is a variation of Cupido, from Ancient Rome, meaning "desire," and this god was also known by the name Amor, or "love." It was thought that Cupid was the son of Venus, the Roman goddess of love.

Eros is at the root of our archetype of erotic love and gives us our concepts of the lover overcome with passion, undone by need, and slain in the heart by love. Our understanding of love in relationships is that it is a passionate, intense emotional bond, solidified by intimacy and connected most deeply by desire.

Is it any wonder that we want to stay in this stage of a relationship? We want that passionate, intense energy. It feeds us and makes us feel alive. This is how we identify love. When that energy fades, we fear that we have fallen out of love.

(continued on page 22)

The History of Love (continued)

Yet much of the early stage of love is about brain chemistry. Our bodies release hormones and brain chemicals that actually make us feel high, and these chemicals promote attachment to each other. Unfortunately, our brains cannot maintain that level of chemical production indefinitely. So, over time, the hormones naturally decrease and our brain chemistry returns to normal. We lose that intense state of desire we call "love." This is when we begin to long for more intensity again.

This is also the phase of our relationship when we have to start working at love. To create passion, we have to make a decision to commit to a deeper connection. The way we do that is through our intimate, erotic connection with our partner.

Better sex often requires more connection, and more intensity.

When you crave more passion in your relationship, you really crave more depth or intimacy. You want a deeper connection to your partner. There is a desire within you to know your partner at a deeper level and to be known at a deeper place. To be connected to another person is a need that both men and women share equally. We fulfill this need through sex. And the more erotic our connection, the more connected we feel with our partner. When our erotic fantasies are fulfilled, we feel a connection with our partner that adds depth and dimension to our partnership.

The Seven Stages of a Relationship

Falling in love is easy to recognize. There are signs and symptoms. For example, we long for our lovers. We feel excited to see them. We think about them often. We desire them sexually. And sometimes we feel like we can't get enough.

Then, when the ardor and thrill of this phase of relationship moves into the more settled stages, we wonder whether we are still "in love." When the signs are different, the highs are not as high, and the attraction is not the same, does this mean that we are no longer in love? And does this mean that the passion is gone?

No. Long-term relationships are not necessarily a death sentence for passion. These phases of partnership are normal and common to everyone. Sexual excitement and eroticism can be part of the life cycle of a relationship if both people are willing to recognize the stages and work on having a long-term, passionate partnership.

Below are the identifiable stages of a relationship.

Romantic love stage. In this stage, we feel alive and awake, and the sex is great. We feel hope and connection. Romantic love generally lasts anywhere from three to twenty-seven months. This is a time of passion and it gives us the bond we need to stay connected during the later stages of love.

The "sweatpants" or comfort stage. At this phase, we feel comfortable in our relationship with our partner and we start to relax. The more familiar we are with each other, the safer we feel, and more of our real selves come to the surface. We also begin to relax the need to focus on our appearance. After the first year, we sometimes start to put on weight and not shave as often, becoming careless about our looks. We also stop worrying about things we might have been concerned about initially and generally settle into the partnership.

The conflict or power struggle stage. In the power struggle phase of a relationship we begin to feel the conflict inherent in every long-term partnership. We become reactive and defensive, trying to protect the love we felt in the beginning of the relationship.

Conflicts happen because we see our partners differently now. After the haze of romantic love has passed, we begin to see our partners without the blur of our projections that we initially saw them through. In the beginning, we see our partners as the people who complete us and make us feel whole. This is because they have personality traits that we ourselves have, but have repressed. We repress those parts of ourselves for lots of reasons, including the feeling that they really aren't effective ways to get love and attention.

For example, if you are a man and you are taught as a child that "big boys don't cry"—a common phrase told to young boys—it is entirely possible that by the time you reach adulthood you will be totally shut off from your capacity to cry when you feel sad. This means that you have repressed the part of yourself that cries.

When you meet a woman and take her to a movie on a date and she cries at the commercials, you might feel overwhelming attraction for her. This is because she has the personality trait that you have repressed. And with her, you can feel whole and complete.

Unfortunately, if you fall in love and marry that woman, eventually her crying will make you crazy! It will feel irritating and annoying, and it will create conflict in your relationship. You will no longer feel attracted to that part of her, but instead will see her crying as distasteful and a way to keep you at a distance instead of attracting your love.

Other reasons that everyday conflicts occur have to do with how we keep score. Men and women are different in the way they relate to the world. Men generally solve problems by retreating and taking time to mull over the problem, coming out of their cave when they have a solution. Women generally talk about their problems until they feel less anxious about them. Men may perceive this as a way to discount their offer of a solution. Women may experience men as "shutting them down" when they don't want to hear about their issues repeatedly.

When we feel conflict in our relationship, our anxiety and stress levels increase and we respond in an almost primitive way. Our brains sense danger and we respond by preparing for a fight, where our systems tense and become ready for physical attack. We might feel we have to defend ourselves or intensify an argument when we feel this response, and unknowingly we heighten the tension for our partner. In many relationships, this stage leads to a withdrawal phase.

Withdrawal stage. Our primitive brain responds to the conflict by going into our defensive behaviors. This is called the fight-or-flight response. We may fight more with our partner when we are scared and feel conflict, or we may withdraw. Our partners react to our defenses by feeling anxious, stressed, and scared. They then respond with their own defenses.

One way people respond to a perceived threat is by going into "flight" mode. This could look like withdrawal. Sometimes your partner may withdraw, to create a sense of safety around him- or herself, to have some space, or to regroup.

Or you or your partner may respond to a power struggle by "freezing." This is the "deer-in-the-headlights" response. This response can look several ways. Your partner may look frozen, be uncommunicative, or freeze, with his mouth open, drool coming out of the corner of his mouth, staring blankly at you while you demand a verbal explanation. You may remain frozen in your pattern, repeating the same things over and over, trying to be heard.

You might forget what you wanted to say, or you might feel foggy or confused during a conflict. This leads to the feeling of "if I don't move, maybe they won't notice me"—camouflage behavior. People who use this defense might try to blend into the background, hoping they won't get hurt, and they will wait out the conflict until the other partner appears to be "done." Then they will breathe a big sigh of relief and "unfreeze."

When conflict goes on for too long, and there is a lot of defensive behavior in both partners, we have a natural tendency to withdraw from each other. We pull back slightly from the relationship, trying to protect ourselves from harm.

We might accept the situation and decide that it's worth staying in for a variety of reasons, including the fact that we still remember the romantic love stage and hope that someday we can get back to that initial feeling. We make a choice, instead of ending the relationship, to go to sleep, sinking into the inevitability of the unhappiness, and focus on outside interests to keep us feeling energized. This begins the "sleep" phase of the relationship.

Sleep stage. In the "sleep" stage of the partnership we may feel at home and comfortable with our partner, but the sexual relationship begins to wane.

Couples at this stage of their relationship may begin to complain about lack of interest in sex, sexual dysfunction, noninitiation, feelings of rejection, abandonment, and resentment toward their partner. (Note: Many physical reasons exist for sexual dysfunction, including blood pressure medications, heart medications, cholesterol medications, menopause, hormonal imbalances, thyroid medication, birth control pills, and antidepressants. See your doctor for physical symptoms of sexual dysfunction, including erectile dysfunction and lack of interest in sex.)

Sex at this point in a relationship may turn into maintenance sex, where you are able to please each other but do so more out of physical need and habit than out of a desire to experience the intensity of your romantic interest in each other. Couples begin to live parallel lives at this stage, creating enough of an individual existence to keep them happy, but not putting the energy into the partnership.

At this point the passion and the eroticism of the relationship begin to get split off. We no longer view our partners as erotic, but as someone to feel safe with. Now we are safe, but we are not fully awake and erotic. We are, essentially, asleep.

Waking up stage. The good news is that there is another stage of a relationship—the "waking up" stage. Sometimes one or both partners recognize that the partnership needs help to return to or begin a new stage of passion and connection. This is the time that many couples come to therapy. One partner recognizes the problem and doesn't want to stay asleep. Both partners remember the "alive" feeling of sexual connection and of being in love. They want to feel energized and passionate again. The process of learning to talk to each other begins.

Learning to explore and share erotic fantasies can create new ways to connect. Connecting can keep a partnership awake and alive for the long term. Before the "waking up" stage of the relationship can begin, we have to take a look at what has happened to our erotic needs along the way.

Love Is in the Longing

New relationships often come with an erotic charge between partners. We don't necessarily feel safe and secure yet, but we may experience an intense sexual feeling, a longing for the other person that happens when we are separated.

We think about our new partners when we are apart from them, and begin to fantasize, guessing about their body parts, which we might not have seen yet, and wondering what sexual positions might feel good with this new person in our lives. Our sexual attraction is created in the longing. It is in the distance between us that we feel desire for the other.

Our experience of romantic love includes a feeling of longing, of missing our loved one. We romanticize the missing of our loved one. Most poetry and love song lyrics are about longing and the intensity of separation. For most of us, this is how we experience falling in love.

As the newness of a relationship wears off, desire for each other seems to decrease and we settle into a nice, safe form of loving that can feel secure, but not always passionate. With familiarity, the longing decreases. We no longer have distance between us. We have found someone to whom we can feel close and connected. This stage of the relationship feels wonderful, safe, warm, and loving. And yet we don't necessarily stay in that same state of bliss we experienced when we were falling in love and longing for connection.

How to Bring Back the Sex You Want— The Next Steps

Margaret Mead, the famous anthropologist, said we have three marriages in our lifetime. The first is for children, the second is for sex, and the third is for companionship. And we can experience all three of those "marriages" in one relationship, or several. Furthermore, we can have a lasting sexual relationship through our child-rearing years, and later through our companionship times.

Sex is a way to feel connected and loving toward our partner. Eroticism can be a physical language in which we express intimacy. It is the closest we can get to our partner on a physical level. It shows trust and openness and can express attraction and affection. Throughout the life span of a relationship, sex can repair hurt, heal grief, bond us after arguments, provide tenderness, comfort us, and help with self-esteem and self-confidence.

Most of all, sex is an expression of love.

We are all looking for love. Love has two components—companionship and erotic connection. Companionship, or "hang-out ability," is what we feel when we enjoy spending time together. Companionship becomes more and more important over time.

The other component of a relationship is eroticism. Eroticism is what keeps the relationship vital and awake and makes us feel sexually connected. Without it, a long-term partner can feel more like a roommate. Working on the eroticism in a relationship is a key element to keeping it vital and alive.

Some couples are willing to give up the sexual part of the relationship because it seems too hard to work at keeping it alive. Communicating about sex, working on the erotic needs of the relationship, and focusing on a healthy partnership where sex is a priority can be a challenge and a commitment.

When there are other priorities like children and work, couples can take their relationship for granted. Being companions can feel easier than working on a sexual connection.

The Need for Honesty

The beginning of this journey to increased erotic connection starts with learning how to talk to each other about sex, as you are learning to do in these exercises. Most of us aren't really honest with our partners about sex.

For example, more than 70 percent of women fake orgasms, according to studies. More and more men are faking it, too. (Men can fake orgasm easily, particularly if they ejaculate inside a woman's vagina. Women take it for granted that if a man says he orgasms that he has indeed ejaculated, regardless of appearance of ejaculate. This can happen more and more as men get older.)

It is sometimes difficult to talk to our partners about our deepest fantasies because erotic needs are many times a part of us that we keep hidden, especially from those we are closest to. Sharing a need or desire that is different than what we have been practicing in our intimate lives can feel threatening to our relationship.

Long-term partnership and intimacy can be reinforced by honest and direct communication about sexual needs. This can happen when we feel free and open enough to share our fantasies with our partner.

Establishing Trust through the Imago Dialogue

We've all heard that an important part of relationships is communication, but why then can't we do it? It seems like most people don't have any problem telling each other what is bothering them or what is lacking in their relationship. It is fairly easy to point out in our partners all of their shortcomings. And many times we repeat this list of complaints, hoping to get our needs met.

In the beginning romantic phase of our relationships we use "appreciation" to get the love we want, and yet later on in the "conflict" phase of a relationship we think we can demand love by telling our partners all the ways in which they are doing it "wrong."

Forcing our partners to give us what we need doesn't work. We have to create a new way of relating to each other. The Imago method of communication does this by providing a safe, structured way to communicate concerns and appreciations. This way of increasing connection allows us to find the passion from the beginning romantic phase of our relationship. It is normal and healthy to crave that erotic connection. But to feel this connection, we need to do the work of communicating intimately, which can help us have that connection and begin to have the sex we really want.

This process is not for the faint of heart. We don't talk about sex easily in our culture. And, interestingly, we talk about sex the least often with the person we are having sex with. Learning the language of intimacy is sometimes, for many couples, a whole new language of love. The language of sex and erotic need is sometimes a difficult and new language to learn.

Talking to each other using words that have been forbidden, dangerous, and illicit can be guilt provoking and feel "bad." Yet this new language can also be a way to add spice and erotic electricity to the relationship, all without even a physical touch.

In this next exercise, you will try to create a safe space to talk about sex, and later explore your fantasies, using words and language that you will grow more comfortable with.

Try this exercise without touching and notice what happens between you and your partner. Can you feel the erotic energy increase? Do you feel yourself blush? Can you feel the pull of the words? Notice what you feel in your body and what you respond to. Try to discuss these feelings and responses with your partner after the exercise.

EXERCISE
Talk Dirty to Me

In this exercise, we will expand on the previous exercise, and take our erotic language skills to a whole new level. This is another great way for couples to create an erotic conversation. You may feel silly, embarrassed, and guilty. All of this is normal and healthy. Do the exercise anyway. You may be pleasantly surprised at how connected you feel to your partner, and how turned on you are when you are through.

(continued on page 32)

(continued)

You will need at least thirty minutes of uninterrupted private time together. Make sure the kids are taken care of, and you have total privacy, so that you will have no fear of being overheard or disrupted. This will help you feel comfortable and safe using whatever language you need to with your partner. Find a quiet place where you can sit comfortably facing each other, close enough so that you can whisper in each other's ear.

In this exercise you will write and share what you write with each other. Make sure you have paper and something to write with and that you can see in the low light of the room. Dark markers or pens work well. Make sure you have a surface to write on that is comfortable for you. A small clock or timer may work if you want to limit the time you both take for the writing portion of this exercise.

You might want to turn down the lights, put on soft music, light some candles, and put on comfortable and sexy clothes. Setting the right mood is a great way to get started, and can help lead to increased passion. Turning down the lights so that there is slightly more darkness in the room can make this exercise easier, but make sure the room is not totally dark. You do not need to be ashamed and hide to do this work. Everything you do here is between loving and safe partners.

Try to stay focused on the exercise for the duration of both sending and receiving.

Step One

Choose who will be the sender and who will be the receiver. The sender is the first one to talk, and the receiver is the first one to listen. The sender will talk and the receiver's only job is to listen and mirror exactly what the sender says. Remember, mirroring means to say back what the sender has said with no other comments.

Step Two

After deciding who will be the sender, both of you should write down ten sexual words. They can be words that describe your or your partner's body parts or they can be words that describe sexual acts. Take five minutes to do this portion of the exercise. If you want to set a timer to remind you both when the time is up, you can do this, or just give each other time to write down the words.

Step Three

After you've done this, senders should say the words quietly to their partners, slowly whispering them in the receiver's ear.

Step Four

Now lean back, make eye contact, and say the words out loud while facing your partner. Remember, giggling is okay.

Step Five

Now say them one more time, and let the receiver mirror each word back, maintaining eye contact.

Step Six

While maintaining eye contact, add an adjective or descriptive word before each word on your list and say them out loud to your partner, who should mirror back after each one.

Examples might be "beautiful vagina" or "hard penis."

Step Seven

Switch roles.

When you are finished with the exercise, discuss with your partner how it felt to do the exercise. How did it feel to say the words? How did it feel to hear the words? How do you feel now?

Talking about sex is not easy, but it is worth it. This type of dialogue can help a partnership that has turned stale become the exciting relationship you crave. It can also take a good relationship and make it hot.

Mirroring, Validating, and Empathizing

Let's review the Imago dialogue, and add more depth to the parts we already know.

Mirroring is simply listening, but in an active way, without inserting our opinion. Mirroring is a way of responding by only repeating what we have heard and "sending" the information back. Giving our partners a chance to say what's on their mind and then mirroring it back allows them to hear what they have said and gives them a chance to change what they meant to say, clarify it, and get to the heart of the matter.

Example:

Sender: "I really appreciate you taking the time to massage my back this morning when we made love."

Receiver: "So what I hear you saying is you really appreciate me taking the time to massage your back this morning when we made love."

Sender: "Well, I really meant that I loved that you made time to touch me in that caring way, since I know we usually are so rushed in the morning."

Receiver: "So, you really loved that I made time to touch you in that caring way, since we are usually so rushed in the morning. Did I get that?"

Sender: "Yes, that's what I meant."

Validating is the second step in the Imago dialogue. This is an important step for both the sender and the receiver. It helps the sender to feel understood, like what they said made sense. The receiver does not have to agree with what the sender has said, but being validated means the receiver has tried to make sense of the sender's experience. The receiver tries to understand the sender's point of view.

Example:

Receiver: "That makes sense to me; I know you really love it when I massage you."

Sender: "Yes, it really helped me to relax and get into the sex today."

Validation is an important part of a dialogue. Many times in a conversation with our partner we feel misunderstood and are not sure our partner really understands us. Sometimes it can feel like we are speaking different languages or that we come from different planets altogether.

The third part of the Imago dialogue is empathy. Receivers imagine what the senders might be experiencing, and try to step into their shoes and understand what the senders are feeling. Understanding our partner's feelings is what creates empathy. This is important when we talk about each other's sexual feelings as well. To be sexually empathic, we have to begin to understand how our partners feel sexually. What might feel good to them, what they might desire, and what might turn them on could be different for them than for us.

If we empathize with their feelings, it doesn't mean we have the same experience as them. It just means we understand what they might be feeling. When we empathize with our partners, we try to imagine feelings and emotions they might be having.

Example:

Receiver: "So I imagine you feel happy and turned on when I massage you first."

Sender: "I do! I get really happy and I feel hot and then I can't wait to make love to you!"

Receiver: "So you get really happy and you feel hot and can't wait to make love to me!"

The Right Time

You can use this dialogue process to go to the next step and talk about your sexual fantasies, as in the following exercise. Again, using this process may feel stilted, goofy, or silly at first, but it will make your partner feel safe and validated. They will feel listened to and understood. And when your partner feels like this, they will be more likely to give you the connection you want. Your communication will feel safer and more comfortable, and ultimately, become easier. In time you will both feel like your needs are finally being met.

As the receiver for your partner, all you need to do is listen and mirror. The only response needed is empathy and validation. You don't need to react to hearing your partner's fantasies by promising to take them into action. All you need to do is hold the space by having the dialogue. Three important things to remember about the dialogue are

- Remember to always ask your partner "Is now a good time to have a dialogue?" Sometimes we set ourselves up for disappointment if our timing is off.

- If the time isn't right, make an appointment. An appointment to have a dialogue about sex is a great idea, because a longer wait time often leads to a greater erotic charge. Also, our partner might need a safer time or space to talk about erotic needs. Make sure your partner can commit to a later date or time.

- And finally, always start your dialogue with an appreciation!

EXERCISE
Exchanging Fantasies

In this exercise, we will take the appreciation exercise and add *validation* and *empathy*. We will create a safe space to talk more specifically about sex. Remember, appreciation is the doorway into a more connected and intimate sex life with your partner.

For this exercise, you will need at least thirty-five minutes of uninterrupted private time together. Find a quiet place where you can sit comfortably facing each other in chairs, on the floor, or on a bed and maintain eye contact for the entire exercise.

You might want to turn down the lights, put on soft music, light some candles, and put on comfortable and sexy clothes. Setting the right mood is a great way to get started, and can help lead to increased passion later on.

Make sure you have nowhere to go after this exercise. Many times it can lead to lovemaking, but do not put pressure on each other to make that happen.

Step One

Start by again sharing appreciations and continuing to mirror each other. This is a basic dialogue skill, and one we will continue to use. This may still feel awkward and a little goofy, but you may now feel safer with this structure. Giggle, squirm, blush, and feel silly—it's all okay.

Try to stay focused on the exercise for the duration of both sending and receiving.

First, choose who will be the sender and who will be the receiver. The sender is the first one to talk and the receiver is the first one to listen.

This exercise may be more difficult than previous exercises. Now you are talking about your sex life, and being very specific. If you are courageous, trust the process, and follow the dialogue structure, you will find that you can stay in the dialogue with your partner without difficulty. You may feel anxious or embarrassed. Don't be afraid to share those feelings with your partner before or after your dialogue.

Senders will "send" over one thing they appreciate about their partner. The receiver will simply mirror back what the sender says. For example:

Sender: "One thing I appreciate about you is how kind you are."

Receiver: "One thing you appreciate about me is how kind I am."

Step Two

Senders will send over one specific thing about your sex life that they like. The receiver will mirror back what the sender says. For example:

Sender: "One thing I appreciate about being in a sexual relationship with you is how open you are to trying new things."

Receiver: "So one thing you appreciate about being in a sexual relationship with me is how open I am to trying new things."

Step Three

Finally, senders will say one thing they may have fantasized about. The receiver will simply mirror back exactly what the sender sends over. For example:

Sender: "One thing I have fantasized about but possibly not shared before is having sex on an airplane with you."

Receiver: "One thing you have fantasized about but possibly not shared before is having sex on an airplane with me."

Step Four

After the senders have sent over all three steps, receivers will validate what they've just heard. Validation means that you share with your partner how it makes sense to you that he or she might be feeling or fantasizing these things. You don't have to agree with those thoughts and fantasies, and you don't have to do them. Hold all those thoughts and ideas for now. Instead, let your partner know you understand where he or she is coming from.

In response to the first three steps in this exercise, validation might sound like this:

Receiver: "So, knowing you the way I know you, it makes sense that you would appreciate my kindness because I know it means a lot to you when people are thoughtful."

Receiver: "It also makes sense that you like how open I am to trying new things because I know you love to experiment."

Receiver: "It also makes sense that you would fantasize about having sex on an airplane because you like to try risky things."

Step Five

After validation, the sender empathizes with the receiver. Showing empathy for our partners goes a long way to helping them feel understood. Empathy does not

(continued on page 38)

mean that you agree with what they are saying or that you are promising to participate in anything. Instead, it shows that you understand their emotional state. Sharing with your partner how you think he or she might feel could sound like this:

Receiver: "I can imagine that if you were to act out your fantasy you would feel excited and turned on. Did I get that feeling?"

Sender: "Yes, and I would also feel loved and appreciated by you."

Receiver: "So you would also feel loved and appreciated by me."

Sender: "You got me."

Now that you have done this exercise, how do you feel? Can you tell your partner what it was like for you? You do not have to disagree, agree, argue, compromise, or commit. Just sit with what you heard. You can ask questions, but try to soak up the appreciation for now, and read on.

A Sample Dialogue

This is a sample of how to use the Imago dialogue. Try following these steps to make it easier to practice the Imago form of communication.

A specific example of the above dialogue might look like this:

Sender: "One thing I appreciate about being partners with you is that you are committed to improving our relationship."

Receiver (mirrors): "So one thing you appreciate about being partners with me is that I am committed to improving our relationship."

Sender: "One thing I appreciate about being in a sexual relationship with you is how attentive you are to making sure I always have an orgasm."

Receiver (mirrors): "So one thing you appreciate about being in a sexual relationship with me is how attentive I am to making sure you always have an orgasm."

Sender: "Yes, and one specific thing you do while we are having sex that I really like is that you squeeze my breasts when you are kissing me."

Receiver (mirrors): "So one specific thing I do while we are having sex that you really like is when I squeeze your breasts when I am kissing you."

Sender: "Yes. And one thing I have fantasized about but never really shared is that you would squeeze my nipples really hard, maybe pinch them, while we are making love."

Receiver (mirrors): "So one thing you have fantasized about that you have never really shared is that you would like it if I would squeeze your nipples really hard, maybe pinch them, while we are making love. Did I get that?"

Sender: "Yes, you got that!"

Receiver (validates): "So, knowing you the way I know you, it makes sense that you would appreciate the way I always make sure you have an orgasm. I know you appreciate my thoughtfulness, and I know you love to have orgasms! Did I get that?"

Sender: "Yes, you got me!"

Receiver (validates): "It also makes sense to me that you would like it when I squeeze your breasts when I kiss you because I know how sensitive your breasts are."

Sender: "Yes."

Receiver (validates): "And it sure makes sense to me that you might have fantasies about me pinching and squeezing your nipples harder because I know when I have played with them in the past it has really felt great to you. Is that right?"

Sender: "Yes! You got me."

If you are having trouble validating, think about your partner and what you know about her. What do you know about her that would make it seem reasonable that she would feel these things? You don't have to understand, but does it make sense to you that your partner would feel these things, knowing her the way you do? How can you relate to these feelings that she has?

(continued on page 40)

A Sample Dialogue (continued)

If your partner is bringing things up that seem totally out of character, or sharing thoughts and fantasies that are shocking to you, it might be hard to validate what she is saying in this exercise. If you are trying to stay in a dialogue with her and really want to make this exercise work for you, it can be a challenge to stay with it. Mirroring what your partner says can help her feel safe to tell you what's really on her mind. She will feel like you are not judging her, and will be more likely to be honest with you in the future about her desires and fantasies.

After mirroring your partner as well as you can, try validating what she said. Can you find something in what she said that makes sense to you?

After validating your partner, try empathizing with her.

Receiver (empathizes): "I can imagine that when you receive those things in bed you feel—*loved, appreciated, safe, cared for, desired, attractive, alive, young, and excited.* Did I get that?"

Receiver (empathizes): "And I can imagine that having those things makes you feel excited and that if you could fulfill that fantasy you would feel really turned on and alive!"

What are some emotions that you imagine your partner might feel now, and that she might feel if she had her fantasy come true? If you were to put yourself in her shoes, what do you think makes sense about the way she might feel? Now check it out with her.

Receiver: "Did I get that?"

Sender: "Yes, I feel that, and I would feel that, and I would also feel sexually fulfilled if I had that fantasy come true."

Receiver: "So I got your feelings, and you would also feel sexually fulfilled if you had that fantasy come true."

Sender: "You got me."

Real-Life Experiences

Let's take a look at a couple who came into a therapy session and used these techniques to improve their sex life. Notice how they use the dialogue and see whether there are ways that you can use their experiences to help you and your partner improve your communication skills.

Alma and Don came into my office to talk about their issues around sexuality and the blocks in their relationship. For many years they had been sexless. They came to therapy to begin the conversation they both wanted to have about sex.

Don's fears about telling Alma his fantasies were deeply rooted in his past. He had always been afraid to talk about sex because in his childhood he had heard from his church and his family that talking about sex was wrong and that anything outside of sex for procreation was a sin.

Don and Alma built up to the following Imago dialogue, which is a good example of a successful exchange. Using the Imago dialogue, Don asked Alma whether she was ready to hear his fantasies.

Don: "Is now a good time to tell you about one of my fantasies?"

Alma: "Yes, now is fine."

Don: "I am nervous to tell you about this, but have always wanted to share this fantasy with you."

Alma: "So you are nervous to tell me about this, but have always wanted to share this fantasy with me. Is that right?"

Don: "Yes. Well, okay, um, please don't judge me, but … "

Alma: "Oh, so you are asking if I would please not judge you."

Don: "Yes. One of my secret erotic fantasies is actually to masturbate in front of you."

Alma did not respond for a moment. Instead of reacting in any way, positively or negatively, she continued to mirror him.

Alma: "So one of your secret erotic fantasies is to masturbate in front of me. Did I get that?"

Don: "Yes, you got it. I guess I have had that fantasy for a long time."

Alma mirrored his words.

Alma: "So what I hear you saying is that one of your fantasies is that you have thought about masturbating in front of me. Is there more?"

Don described in detail what his deepest and most hidden fantasies were about masturbating for her.

Slowly, as the process continued, Alma was able to hear what Don described, and why he felt the feelings he did. He described his fears about sharing these thoughts with her. He talked about feeling ashamed of his thoughts.

Don: "I don't think it's wrong, but part of me feels like that should be private. I want you to know that I love you and want to share this with you."

Alma: "Oh, so part of you thinks that masturbation should be private, but you don't really think it's wrong. You also want me to know that you love me and want to share this with me."

Don talked about his fears and his childhood prohibition against masturbation. He wondered if he was going to break their marital bond. Alma listened and simply mirrored back, always asking:

Alma: "Is there more?"

Don: "Yes. I was thinking that if we took this fantasy into action, I would want you to do it too, in front of me. Maybe we could do it together, at the same time. That would really be exciting for me, and I would see what you like."

Alma mirrored Don's fantasy, without agreeing or disagreeing. She encouraged Don, simply by staying in the process, to talk through all of his fears and insecurities. She validated his feelings, while not necessarily agreeing with him.

Alma: "I know you have always had a lot of curiosity about a lot of things. So, it makes sense to me that you would wonder about masturbation. I understand that you have had fantasies that might be different than mine. You are a separate person than me."

She understood that as a couple they are differentiated (two different people). Just like Don had different appetites for foods than she did, Alma recognized that he could have different sexual fantasies as well. This did not threaten his love for her.

Her ability to express understanding, regardless of how hard it may have been for her to hear his fantasy, made Don feel safe and secure in their relationship. He felt he could tell her anything. He began to cry in the session, and told Alma he had never felt closer to her.

Using empathy, she tried to guess at his feelings.

Alma: "I can imagine that telling me this fantasy was embarrassing for you, but also that it made you feel relieved, and maybe a little turned on."

Don: "Yes, and I also feel a lot of love for you because you listened to me without judging me."

Alma: "So you also felt love for me because I listened to you without judging you."

Notice that Alma never agreed or disagreed to fulfill Don's fantasy. She simply allowed Don to talk to her freely, and really listened to him express his need.

They agreed that they would continue to explore Don's fantasies. This showed generosity and open-mindedness and made Don feel more secure about his sexuality. Don's gratitude and love for Alma dramatically improved for many sessions after this.

As a result of talking about Don's fantasy, Alma was able to talk about her fantasies, and share with Don erotic thoughts she had. She had never been honest about them because she was afraid Don would reject her if she did. This shame is deeply rooted in childhood, and can interfere with the ability to share erotic needs with our partners.

Adding Risk to Your Relationship

3

All of us want to feel safe and secure in our lives, and marriage and committed partnerships help us to feel that way.

Unfortunately, committed partnerships and marriages still last only about 50 percent of the time, with divorce rates changing little over the past fifty years. Yet, even with such a high rate of divorce, we still seek out marriage as an institution. People are waiting longer to get married, marrying at later ages, and choosing to live together first, but still marrying. More and more, we are marrying a second, and sometimes even a third, time. We still want partnerships, despite knowing that long-term relationships can sometimes lead to the demise of passion and erotic energy in those relationships.

It would seem that the longer we are connected to someone in a safe and secure relationship, the more honest and open we could be about our sexual needs. There would seem to be a connection between long-term partnerships and good sex. And yet, after about ten years of marriage or partnership, many couples complain that they feel "out of love" and no longer feel the passion they once felt.

Splitting Off Sexual Needs

When we are first dating, sex can be hurried or frenetic. The rush adds to the excitement. An element of getting caught can feel thrilling. The mile-high club (having sex on an airplane), elevator sex, or sex in unusual places where there is the possibility of being seen creates a feeling of excitement. The danger makes sex feel erotic.

Because erotic energy feels "dangerous," it can also feel exciting. But keeping the excitement alive is difficult. Our need for exciting and stimulating sex is normal. But after couples have been together for a while, they fear that talking about their erotic needs can corrupt the "safety" of the long-term relationship. So, in actuality, over time it becomes more difficult to talk about what we really want.

Before children come along, we may find that in our early relationship we enjoy long, leisurely weekends of erotic juiciness. Without children we have fewer constraints and lots of uninterrupted time to act out our fantasies. But after we have children, we split off our sexual needs, or bury them, hoping to take them out again when the kids are older, or when we are less tired.

Some of the ways we split off the sexuality from our relationship can include things like looking at pornography or visiting porn sites, having phone sex, chatting on the Internet, or having an affair. Or we can simply close down our sexual needs, splitting them off into a compartment within us, shutting down our sexuality. In some ways, couples can feel that these behaviors keep them in the relationship. It is a way to justify getting their needs met, and keeping the relationship at home safe and secure. They don't have to bring in any of their erotic needs, thereby keeping the home bond sacred and pure.

If we are in a partnership to feel safe and secure, and erotic sex is dangerous and forbidden, then being safe and secure certainly feels antithetical to passion. But splitting off our erotic needs does not help us be closer to our partner, and it doesn't help us get the sex we really want. This is the dichotomy of marriage.

Taking the Next (Risky) Erotic Step

One way to bring the excitement of "forbidden" sexuality into a relationship is to add an element of "practiced spontaneity," or *risk*. In other words, practicing spontaneous ways to keep the sexual relationship alive and vital can recharge the partnership. Ironically, spontaneity can be part of our relationship if we focus on a plan to put it there.

Ironically, spontaneity can be part of our relationship if we focus on a plan to put it there.

In the early stages of a relationship you may have found that the times when you were spontaneous and took risks were your hottest sexual moments. These more risky experiences may have come after a period of not seeing each other for a while. Maybe the times you were apart were the times that you felt a romantic longing for your lover, and perhaps fantasized about what it would be like when you were together again. Maybe you thought about what you wanted to do to your lover the next time you were in bed together. Fantasy and distance can create great erotic energy.

Talking on the phone, for example, is one way to recreate the feeling of that erotic longing. Talking on the phone can feel intimate and far away at the same time. Having sexy phone conversations can add erotic excitement to an already familiar relationship, making it feel young and passionate again.

The other added benefit of talking sexy on the phone is that because there is no eye contact there is a natural distance that is created between you and your partner. This can help those who are naturally more shy or reticent to say things in person. The phone allows for erotic freedom and can be a safe way for you to practice saying things out loud, including sexy things that you want to do to your partner. It can sometimes be easier to share these ideas when you don't have to look at your partner while saying them. Telling your partner on the phone the sexy things you want to do when you get home is great practice for what you can say later, in person.

The following exercise will build on the dialogue skills you learned in the earlier chapters and incorporate some sexier, and maybe even racier, language. Because you will have this conversation over the phone, the safety and distance will add an erotic element that will give you room to take some risks in what you say to each other.

By now you have a new form of communication, the Imago dialogue. You can tell your partner what you want, and all he has to do is listen. He can listen actively by mirroring, validating, and empathizing. You will continue building on this format throughout the book, creating a safe structure to talk about your erotic thoughts and fantasies.

So take risks! Do the exercise and use the sexiest language you can imagine. What words can you come up with that might make your partner blush? Use them! What words describe things you want to do? Will they make you blush? Go ahead… no one will see because you're on the phone!

EXERCISE
Phone Sex

For this exercise, you will need at least ten minutes of uninterrupted private time to call your partner on the telephone. Find a quiet place where you can comfortably make the call, where you know you will not be interrupted or overheard.

This call should be a surprise, so try to call your partner at a time when he or she is not expecting it. It works best if you call during a challenging time in the day when it is hard for your partner to talk openly—when your partner is at work or otherwise occupied. This will increase the tension and the feeling of erotic risk. (Make sure you are not truly putting your partner's job at risk by doing this, if the job entails recorded phone calls, etc.)

As in the previous exercises, we will be sharing and then mirroring. This is a basic dialogue skill and one we will use for many of the other exercises to come. Although you may have practiced it, you might still feel uncomfortable with the slow pace that this creates in your "conversation." See if you can appreciate the slower pace of the dialogue and notice how it brings you closer to your partner, allowing you to appreciate each word and nuance of emotion in what he or she is saying to you.

The words you use on the phone with your partner may feel awkward and forced. That's okay; say them anyway. Let the exercise feel awkward for now. Practicing erotic conversation is a great way to grow toward having better sex!

It doesn't matter if you call first thing in the morning or right before you get home. The earlier you call the more the tension will build toward the moment when you are together again. You can call once in a day or five times. During your call, try to allow your partner to really hear what you have to say, and leave enough room and mystery to think and fantasize about what will happen when the two of you get home.

Step One

Call your partner on the telephone. Tell her in detail what you are planning to do to her when she gets home tonight.

For example, you might have a fantasy of undressing your wife when she gets home. If you are calling her at work, you might say, "Hi, honey, I've been thinking about you," and then ask her, "can you just mirror that back for me?"

(If she can't mirror you—either because of her work environment or another reason—ask her whether she can stay on the phone with you, and if so, ask her to mirror you internally.)

Step Two

Continue the dialogue over the phone, taking your time, and relaying the smallest and most intimate details about how you plan to undress her when she comes home.

Listen while she mirrors you. She may have to repeat it a couple of times until she gets it. You might have to send it over again if she didn't get it all. Then tell her more.

Tell her, "I can't wait to sit you down on the edge of the bed and slowly slide off your shoes." Let her mirror you.

Tell her how you will then "slowly and very carefully pull each stocking off of her thighs." Then ask her to mirror that.

Then tell her, "And then I am going to touch your smooth legs and soft thighs. And I can't wait to pull your panties off very slowly, down your thighs and off of your legs ... "

And ask her to mirror you. She may be breathless by now, or feel silly and giggle. She might feel surprised at how uncomfortable it is to feel so erotic. Keep telling her intimate details of what you are thinking of doing. This may seem awkward and uncomfortable, particularly if you have never used this kind of language before.

Remember, you are on the phone, and she can't see you blush! Keep describing in detail what you want to do to her.

"And then I will slide my hands up your legs and very slowly touch you between your legs with my fingers to see how wet you are."

Then ask her if she's wet just listening to you! And then ask her to mirror you back.

(continued on page 50)

(continued)

Step Three

Finally, when you feel she has had enough, or if you want to leave her wanting more, you can ask her to validate and empathize for you. Say, "So, knowing me the way you know me, does it make sense that this is what I am thinking about?"

And let her tell you why it makes sense to her that you would want these things. It might sound like, "Yes, it makes sense that you would want to do these things. I know you love my legs and you would love to take my stockings off and touch my thighs. And I know you love it when I am wet for you, so I can imagine that you would love to put your hand on me to feel that wetness and how turned on I am."

Then you might ask her to empathize with you, or imagine your emotions. It might sound like, "And what do you imagine I might feel if we did all these things?"

And see whether she can guess your feelings. If she gets them, then just say, "Yes, you got me."

If there are other feelings as well, you can add them.

"Yes, you got me and I would also feel totally turned on, crazy for you, hot, and madly in love."

Step Four

Hang up and get ready! At this point you can decide how long you will take to get home, or to meet your partner. You might take your time, building the tension, and calling a few more times to add to your fantasy list. Or you might hang up the phone and rush home, to fulfill your fantasy with your partner.

Remember that going home might not seem as risky and exciting as being on the phone did. If you have children, make sure there is a babysitter or someone to take care of them for a few hours. If there are chores to be done or things like taking care of pets, etc., make sure you take care of what you need to and find time to focus completely on your partner and your relationship. You both deserve to have this time to yourselves, and to take your phone sex conversation one step further!

Adding Excitement to Sex

Remember, eroticism is a way to express love. It is through connection with each other that we find the ultimate union and can experience love in physical form, the ultimate sensual experience.

Sometimes we forget this. Or we feel torn about our erotic needs. This is because erotic fantasies are often loaded with anticipation and a feeling of being "bad" or "naughty." This feeling can add an element of excitement to sex. Erotic fantasy is often more edgy than the sex we have in real life because we may imagine things we have been taught are wrong or illicit and have erotic fantasies about them. Examples might include fantasies about having sex in a public place or masturbating in front of our partner.

The exercises in this chapter and the next one will help you explore the "naughty" part—the sexual and erotic self inside that longs to come out and play. That part of us wants expression, and it yearns to feel free and open to express its "bad" side. If we can be "naughty" in our relationship, with someone we feel safe with, then we can have the best of both worlds. We have safety, and we have risk. Eroticism can be explored freely when we feel safe, but only if we feel safe enough to take the risk to be "bad."

EXERCISE
When Being Bad Is Oh... So Good

In this exercise, you will share your memories and thoughts with your partner after you have written them down, so you will need a piece of paper or a journal. Building on the Imago dialogue, you will mirror what your partner shares, which will help him to mirror you when you talk about what you have written.

Remember, there is no right or wrong way to do this exercise. This is the beginning of practicing a new way of relating to your partner. It may feel awkward or embarrassing at first. That's always okay. Taking a risk sometimes means doing things we aren't comfortable with at first.

For this exercise, you will need at least thirty to sixty minutes of uninterrupted private time together. You will need a quiet place where you can first sit comfortably and write for about ten minutes. Next, you will need twenty to fifty minutes to dialogue with your partner.

(continued on page 52)

(continued)

Find a comfortable place to sit facing your partner, either in chairs or on a bed. Try to see if you can maintain eye contact for the entire exercise.

Step One

Using your journal and a pen, take a moment and remember something "naughty" or "bad" you did when you were first having sex with your partner. Did you have sex in a place where there was a risk of getting caught? Did you try new positions that you normally wouldn't perform? What kinds of risks did you take? Was there anything you did that made you feel particularly erotic at the beginning of your sex life together?

Write down any "naughty" things you can think of.

Step Two

Think about what "naughty" or "bad" thing you want to do to your partner right now. Remember, your idea of "naughty" may be different than your partner's. That's okay. Just write down something that makes you feel "bad" when you fantasize about doing it now with your partner.

Don't worry about what your partner will think or say—the receiver's only job is to mirror you. Your partner doesn't have to agree to do it, or have a conversation about it. Right now we are just practicing the early parts of the Imago dialogue.

When you have written down one "naughty" sexual thing you want to do with your partner now, let him know that you are done and ready to dialogue.

Step Three

Choose who will be the sender and who will be the receiver. The sender will "send" over what he has written about remembering something naughty from early in the relationship.

The receiver will simply repeat, or mirror, what the sender says.

An example might be the following:

Sender: "I remember having sex with you in the back of my convertible, outside on the street in front of your house."

And the receiver would simply say back, maintaining eye contact: "So, you remember having sex with me in the back of your convertible, outside on the street in front of my house. Is there more?"

The sender can say "yes" and send more or "no" and stop there. After the receiver has mirrored, the sender switches and becomes the receiver.

Now that you have shared your memories and fantasies with each other, how do you feel? Can you tell your partner what it was like to hear those things? Try not to judge what you heard, or disagree, or argue about them. You can ask questions, but try to just be curious for now. If it feels comfortable, move on to having that naughty experience! Make sure your partner wants to and is ready to take this experience into action.

If you are both intrigued and want to try this new (or old) risky behavior, then go for it. Or make a date to make your fantasy come true!

Just knowing that the time is coming when you will have fun and do something "bad" will build your erotic energy and excitement. You may feel more attracted to each other. It might even remind you of the old days—when you were first in love.

An Appointment with Passion

Another way to increase the readiness for passion is to make a date for sex! Some couples object to this because they feel like it takes the spontaneity out of the relationship, and therefore depletes the passion.

Actually, many times it does the opposite. If we know that sex is coming on Saturday night, we can plan for it! Remember, eroticism is in our minds—it is in our fantasy life. If we have some lead time, we can begin to use our imagination and our fantasies to create sexual tension, and by the time our "sex date" comes along, we have been looking forward to it for a while.

If you think back to when you were dating and had plans to meet, it is entirely possible that you knew you would have sex play that night. You were prepared in your mind and in your imagination. The anticipation added an element of erotic connection to the night. Sex dates do the same thing. They allow time for physical preparation, including waxing, shaving, buying lingerie, taking special baths, etc. They can also increase the time available to plan special surprises or appreciations for your partner prior to the date.

If you can schedule a sex date every week, on the same night, it can bring many benefits to your relationship. For example, even though one or both of you may not be in the mood for sex, a sex date means that you do it anyway. And the more you "do it anyway" the more you want to do it. Sex hormones increase the more sex you have. And the more your body and your mind get used to the idea and the rhythm of the regularly scheduled sex date, the more you will naturally anticipate the sex.

For women in particular, this long lead time can lead to a slow buildup, which corresponds with their sexual plateaus that physically lead up to orgasm. Women need to build up slowly until their bodies are ready for orgasm. Having several days lead time every week can really contribute to a buildup of passion before the date.

The sex date also adds an element of respect to the sexual aspect of the partnership. It makes sex a priority. It's what we mean when we say "relationships take work." Work means scheduling, making sex a priority, and doing it even if you don't feel like it. The great part of working on your sex life and scheduling sex dates is that you get to make your passionate partnership a priority in your life. Date night becomes more important than other things that might creep up in your schedule. This gives your partner the very clear message that your partner is important to you, and that a healthy and passionate sex life is a priority!

A Date with Desire

Ken and Dara, a couple in their late thirties, used their date night to revive their sex life, after their three kids and both their jobs had taken a toll on their energy and enthusiasm for each other.

Neither of them wanted sex to go to the bottom of the list, and yet after the kids and sleep, it began to lose its appeal. Without it, they both felt disconnected from each other, and frustrated. They argued more, and felt more conflict in their relationship. Because they knew that the erotic part of the relationship would keep them alive and connected, and they wanted to stay passionate toward each other, they created a date night, on Friday nights, every other week.

They got a sitter and rented a hotel room in their neighborhood. They had take-out food brought in, ate dinner in bed, and planned a different fantasy to act out each date night. One night they would watch soft porn movies on the hotel television. One night they dressed up in costumes and acted out a role-play fantasy. One night they lit candles and gave each other long, sensual massages.

They found that they both began anticipating their Friday night sex dates with glee and a secret determination to keep those nights a sacred part of their relationship. Both of them kept the nights a priority, working around babysitting difficulties, illness, money, and weather conflicts. They agreed that those nights got them through the early years of child rearing and kept their relationship alive and passionate, even adding a new level of eroticism for both of them that they had not known existed.

For date night, pick nights and times that are realistic, even if they still challenge your schedule a little. Some challenge is okay. Remember, date nights mean making sex and passion a priority. When you have your date nights picked out, mark them on your calendar… in pen.

Decide where you will go and what you will do. If you have kids, get a babysitter. Plan your outfit. Use your imagination to add any unusual or special elements to the night. Do you need candles? Do you need a blanket to have sex outside? Do you need to make a reservation? How can you surprise your partner on date night, remembering fantasies he or she may have shared with you in the previous exercises? Now have fun!

When Erotic Needs Split Off from the Relationship

When we are in a long-term partnership, and grow past the romantic love phase, it seems like the sex begins to change. Our passion for each other seems to wane. Our own sexuality might feel different. We are still physically driven to have sex with our partners but might find the frequency diminishes, and sometimes the emotional desire to be close to our partners decreases as well.

When this happens, our natural "Eros" needs, our passion, begins to split off from the relationship. Because our erotic needs are normal and natural, they have to go somewhere—they don't just disappear. If we don't work on getting our erotic needs met and dealing with these issues and challenges, we will act out some of our frustrations and our relationships may suffer.

Our needs can indeed be met when we understand what happened to them and what we can do with our partners to help feel erotic and alive again.

As noted before, the safer your relationship, the more your erotic needs may become split off from the partnership. This is not a sign that the relationship isn't going to work—it may instead indicate that you are invested in its survival, but just haven't figured out a way to integrate your erotic needs within your safe relationship.

There are specific ways to do this, and the exercises in this book can help.

The following issues explain the reasons that our erotic needs get shut off or split off from our relationships. As you read about them, try to identify whether any of these apply to you or your partner.

Madonna/Whore Complex

The Madonna/whore complex is a projection of roles or archetypes onto women that applies only to part of who the complete, sensual woman truly is. Women in our culture are often viewed as either the "Madonna" or the "whore."

This belief has roots in our most sacred stories. Mary Magdalene and the Virgin Mary are examples of this split. When women give birth to children, they become the "mother"—a pure symbol of wholesomeness and nurturing. They are viewed as pure and untouchable.

Sometimes this view of their lover as the "mother" makes it difficult for men to see their partners as the sexual and erotic women they once were. Now that they have borne children, men can see their partners as too "mother-like" to feel sexy toward them.

In our culture, we see women as "bad girls" if they want sex and "good" if they don't. Many women have difficulty integrating the sexual parts of themselves because they feel "bad" if they want sex. And being a mom and wanting sex can be very confusing for women. So they compartmentalize; that is, they put away their erotic needs in a little box deep down inside "until the kids are older." Being a mom and being sexy at the same time are hard roles to balance. It is hard to make macaroni and cheese during the day for the children and then go upstairs and put on the sexy garter belt at night!

When men start to see their partners as "mom," and not the women whom they have sex with, the erotic energy may dissipate. Sometimes men feel torn about their attraction for their partner when they are in this role.

EXERCISE
Exploring the Madonna/Whore Woman

For this exercise, you may need several nights, or dates. Find time when the kids are taken care of and you will not be interrupted. You will need a day or an evening where there is no pressure and you can take your time.

Know that for some women, these role-plays may bring up difficult feelings or emotions, but they will also bring out joy and sexual celebration.

You can divide this exercise and use different role-plays on different date nights. Be the good girl on one date, and the bad girl on the next. Keep your partner guessing!

Step One
Write down all the ways that you are a good mother or a good nurturer if you are not a mother.

Step Two
Now write down all of the ways that you a sexy, erotic woman.

Step Three
Share your list with your partner.

Step Four
Now play with the idea of "good girl/bad girl." How can you have sex as the "good girl" and how can you set up erotic play as the "bad girl"? For example, as the good girl, try wearing white, lacy lingerie, and become your softest, most nurturing and loving self. Make love with the lights off, in the missionary position, and see how sexy you can make that for your partner. Whisper in his ear, "I'm a good girl, you are doing such good things to me!" or maybe pretend to be nervous, scared, and virginal. Whisper in your partner's ear, "I am so scared… please don't hurt me … ."

And see whether your partner can whisper in your ear, "I love that you are a good girl, and I will be oh so gentle … ."

Step Five
As a bad girl, try dressing in black, in leather, and baring lots of skin. Have sex with your partner on top, and talk firmly in his ear as you are doing it—"I am a bad, bad girl, and I am going to do anything I want to you!" Play with that powerful, sexy self, and feel the bad girl come out to take control!

The Hunger for Sex versus Food

Women in general have a hard time recognizing what they want and asking for it. Frequently, women have been taught that hungering for sex is not okay.

Because we grow up in a culture where being thin is more important than being healthy, most adult women have been on at least two diets in their lifetime. Dieting often means denying physical hunger. It also means that many women who have been dieting most of their adult life have gotten out of touch with their bodies and the body's natural signal for hunger. Learning to listen to the body and its signals and desires can then be difficult.

Women sometimes experience their sexual needs as a feeling of hunger. When they feel a stirring in their body, they might not understand that this is a sexual stirring. They don't know how to identify what their hunger really is. This may be in part because girls are not taught what to do with their sexual desire.

Girls who begin dieting when they are young learn to turn off the small voice inside that tells them they are hungry. How many times do women stand in the kitchen in front of the cabinets, looking for something to fill a craving? Sometimes nothing seems to satisfy because the craving isn't always for food. It might actually, sometimes, be for sex.

Women may not recognize what it feels like to have a physical craving for sex. They have not been taught to listen to their hunger for sex, or to recognize their body's signals.

For women, it is easier to repress their sexual needs or turn them into self-destructive acts like compulsive eating or starving. Are women trying to prove how strong they are by not listening to any of their body's signals? Or are they just cut off from what they are really craving?

Because women have not been taught to recognize when they want sex, they don't really know how to ask for it. If they cannot recognize the desire for sex, they cannot recognize what kind of sex they want. And they therefore can't ask for it!

EXERCISE
Recognizing What Your Body Hungers for

This exercise is about increasing the awareness of your body. Keep focused until you can identify all the different feelings in your body.

For this exercise you will need at least fifteen minutes of uninterrupted time. A comfortable place to sit or lie down will help you get in touch with your physical sensations.

Step One

Find a way to sit or lie down that allows you to feel all the parts of your body. Close your eyes and take at least three deep breaths. Try and breath all the way down into your belly, softening your center to let in as much air as you can, and then making your exhalation longer than your inhalation.

Notice how your body relaxes as you breathe deeply.

Step Two

Start at your feet and notice what your feet are feeling. Are they tired, sore, or cold? Do they feel warm and relaxed?

Now move up your legs and notice what your legs feel like. Can you feel tingling or energy in your legs? You can touch your legs with your hands if you want, and feel the shape of them as they lead you to your center.

Now move up to your genitals and your reproductive organs. Can you feel what your genitals are experiencing right in this moment? Do you feel tingling or tightness? Relaxation?

Try to identify words in your mind that describe this whole area. Words might be "sexy, relaxed, tight, wet, tense," etc. Try to experience all the sensations there. Use your hands there to explore the sensations and think about what you are feeling.

Now move up your body through your back and belly. Notice how they feel, and move your awareness up to your chest. Do you feel yourself breathing? Do you feel aroused? Are your nipples responding to your thoughts? To your touch?

Now move your awareness up to your neck and face and hair. Notice how your face and neck respond to your breathing and to your touch.

(continued on page 60)

(continued)

Try to be aware of how you are feeling in this moment. Breathe deeply and notice where in your body you feel sensation. Are you hungry? Tired? Warm or cold? Do you feel aroused or stimulated?

Now you have a language to recognize your body and its responses. Keep this in mind the next time you are wondering what (or whom) you are hungry for.

"Parentifying" Our Partners

Another aspect of partnership that interferes with sexuality is the need for *dependence*. To some extent, we as humans are all dependent on each other. And yet the healthiest relationships include a sense of "differentiation," or the recognition that our partners are separate from us, and might not always want the same things as us.

Sometimes we treat our partners as extensions of ourselves. We assume that if we are hungry, they are hungry. If we are tired, then they must be tired. If we want to have sex, then our partner must as well!

However, our partners have their own erotic needs and interests. We make assumptions that if our partners loved us they would just "know" what we wanted—in the relationship and in bed. But this is not true! We cannot psychically divine what our partners want unless they tell us.

Living with a partner brings a set of issues unique to cohabitation. We "parentify" our partners by projecting onto them our needs. In other words, if you chase your partner around, nagging him to pick up his socks, then he will begin to see you as a parent figure, and not as a partner. If you boss your partner around, or try to have control over her behaviors, then your partner will experience you as parental. This means she probably will not want to have sex with you! Parentifying desexualizes the relationship.

In addition, if we add children to the family, our priorities change. Our need to create a safe environment for kids becomes paramount. We want safety and security for our children, so the heightened need for security in the house-hold supersedes the need for eroticism. The childbearing years are, for most couples, the hardest time of the relationship. These years may coincide with the conflict phase and stress the partnership to its limits, and with good reason.

Having kids is very stressful. The job of being a parent is physically and emotionally exhausting. Sometimes the end of the day means the finish line for parents of young children, when the need to sleep feels more important than having sex with the coparenting partner.

Trusting that this is a phase of the relationship is important. This time will pass, and the kids will grow up. The time for passionate connection will return. Meanwhile, working on that continued connection in your relationship is very important.

EXERCISE
Hot Night Out

This exercise is different from date night. This is a one-time night out that is expressly for your stress relief and to remember that you are both adults and that there is more to your relationship than being parents. Remembering that there is a grown-up connection between you can revitalize a parenting relationship that may have become desexualized and exhausted.

Make this a special night. Make it an escape. Make it a hot night out that you take for a treat. And do it as often as you think you need to restore that feeling of passion in your relationship. Get a babysitter for an evening.

Plan on the kind of sex you want to have on your night out. Are you craving a relaxed, sensual night, where you spend lots of time on massage, talking, and taking a long hot bath together?

Maybe you need to have more edgy sex to break free of your roles as parents. Tying each other up with silk scarves or using a silk scarf as a blindfold can be a fun way to add some excitement to your hot night out (later exercises will help you explore these types of erotic elements in more detail). For now, decide on one element that you will add to your night. The following are some suggestions: bring along massage oil, order or rent pornography, order room service and feed each other fruit or other sensual foods, or take a bath together.

If you have an overnight babysitter, enjoy a night's sleep together!

The Shame that Keeps Us from Going "There"

There may be a deep erotic well inside of you that you find you have trouble accessing. You might sense that you are a passionate person who wants to explore many aspects of your sexuality, but are not sure how to do that.

Shame contributes to the splitting off of sexuality and erotic needs. Appreciation can go a long way to helping your partner heal from shame.

We all have parts of ourselves that we hold back. Sometimes we might feel embarrassed about our needs, or our curiosities. We might even feel ashamed of what we feel or want. Shame can keep us from feeling free and alive. Working through that shame, with the help of your partner, can free passionate energy and allow more intensity into your erotic life. So how does shame happen?

Webster's Dictionary defines shame as "a painful emotion caused by consciousness of guilt, shortcoming, or impropriety. A condition of humiliating disgrace or disrepute. Something that brings censure or reproach. Something to be regretted."

Shame is a learned feeling, and it comes from many places. It has its roots in our religious organizations, in our government's desire to control sexual practices and relationships, and through our own fears that we are somehow different than everyone else.

We also receive messages from our parents about what sex is about. Can you think of what your parents taught you about sex? What is one word your parents might have used to describe sexuality when you were growing up?

What is one word your parents would have used to describe their own sexual relationship, if you could guess? How do you think these feelings and beliefs affect you now as an adult? How do you think they affect you as a sexual person in a relationship?

Shame contributes to the splitting off of sexuality and erotic needs. Our need for sex and passion does not disappear, it just splits off. It can split off into pornography, internet relationships, affairs, sexual addiction of all kinds, and other problems. When there is no appropriate channel for our erotic needs, the energy has to go somewhere. That split-off energy sometimes has no outlet when there is intense shame involved.

The hard part of the sexual relationship when there is shame is that it separates us from our partner. How do we talk to our partner about our sexual and erotic needs when we have shame about them? Shame happens when one's fantasies are imagined to be harmful to another. When we feel shame it can be hard to share what we really want.

However, research shows that people are much more open to hearing what we say when we start with an "appreciation."

Many times in the later stages of our relationship we fail to mention the positives and start nagging our partners about what makes us unhappy. We criticize and let our partner know how unhappy we are. But we don't tell them what we appreciate.

Behaviorists tell us that to extinguish a negative behavior we should ignore it, not exert pressure to change it. To get more of a positive behavior we should appreciate it!

Reminding our partners of what we appreciate about them will create more of that behavior. This works when we talk to our partners about our sex life. When we want to have a conversation about our erotic needs, the last thing we want to do is shame our partner. We want to build up their confidence in themselves so that they are more likely to respond to us in a positive way.

Appreciation can go a long way toward helping your partner heal from shame. And it can also be a way to feel safe to share the things you want in a sexual relationship.

As you try this next exercise, remember what you have done in the previous exercises, and how it felt to have your partner mirror back everything you said. You will, by now, have had an experience of really being heard and seen by your partner. Knowing how this has helped you to feel safe and connected, you can give this experience to your partner to help him feel those things as well.

EXERCISE

Appreciating Your Partner Sexually

This exercise includes writing and sharing. Have something to write on and a pen or pencil. You will write a short list and then share what you wrote with your partner. Have a comfortable place to write and enough light to see.

Find a comfortable place to sit or lie down for at least thirty minutes. Make sure the kids are taken care of and you have total privacy. Create an atmosphere of sensuality by turning the lights low, lighting candles or incense, and turning on soft music. Allow yourself to make eye contact with your partner, sitting close enough so he or she can see your eyes, and reach out to hold hands.

Know that this exercise may make you feel embarrassed, or even bring up some shame. You might feel awkward or silly. This may make you want to run away, or hide. Take a deep breath when you feel this way. Notice how your pulse quickens and your heart races. Remember that his happens during sex, too, and can be an exciting and sexy part of the exercise. It's okay to feel nervous. Try to stay with your feelings and honor them.

Step One

First, take out your paper and pencil and think about the things you appreciate that your partner does in bed. List three of these things.

Step Two

Next, list three things you would like more of.

Step Three

When you are both ready, decide who will be the sender first and who will be the receiver. Share your answers with your partner. For example:

Sender: "So, one thing I really appreciate that you do in bed is give great oral sex."

Receiver (mirrors): "So one thing you really appreciate that I do in bed is give great oral sex."

Repeat until all three things have been mirrored.

Step Four

Validate and empathize with one another. For example:

Receiver (validating): "So, it makes sense that you would like the way I perform oral sex because you are really turned on when I do it, and I imagine that when I do that it makes you feel really excited because it always makes you orgasm."

Step Five

Switch. Receivers become the senders and send three things they appreciate that their partner does in bed. The receiver mirrors these three statements, then validates and empathizes with them.

Step Six

Repeat the process, with the senders sending over the three things they would like more of, and with the receivers mirroring them after each statement, followed by validation and empathy.

Notice what happens when you are through with sharing this exercise. What do you feel toward your partner? How are you feeling about what you shared? If you are feeling any embarrassment, share it with your partner now using the Imago dialogue. For example:

Sender: "I am embarrassed about admitting that I like oral sex so much."

Receiver: "So you are embarrassed about admitting that you like oral sex so much. Is there more?"

Just mirror and ask whether there is more until the embarrassment has been talked through. Now switch if the receiver has any embarrassment about what the sender shared.

Notice what happens now that you have shared your embarrassments. What do you feel toward your partner? How are you feeling about what you shared? What are you feeling in your body? Do you feel any sexual stirrings or physical longings for your partner?

The Difference in Arousal Levels

Most women have a long lead time when it comes to passion. Men need to know that if they want to have sex on a Saturday, they should probably start on a Wednesday!

This is because women have many arousal plateaus that they need to go through before they reach their peak. Before they ultimately are ready to orgasm, they need to be aroused for a while. Most men, however, have one arousal plateau. They need to be touched, preferably directly on their penis, to create a peak physical arousal.

The good news for women is that because their arousal levels rise slowly, they also come down slowly, which is what enables women to have multiple orgasms. What men need to know about women's long lead time is that they need to start foreplay days ahead to prepare a woman emotionally and physically for sex.

One way that men can prepare women for sex is to connect physically before an actual night of sex. Coming up behind your partner and kissing her on the neck unexpectedly, and then walking away, without expectation, adds an element of sexiness without pressure. Phone calls and text messages that tell her you are thinking of her in erotic ways, notes left under her pillow, or whispered fantasies in her ear in the car while she's driving are all good ways to lead up to a hot erotic night that might not officially begin for several days.

EXERCISE
Sensual Full-Body Contact

One way to begin to build up passion is to enjoy physical contact in a new way. Feeling the body of your partner and being mindful of how it feels against you can increase sexual feelings for each other.

For this exercise, you will need at least forty minutes of uninterrupted time together. In this exercise you will be totally naked with each other. There may be some awkwardness or discomfort at first, but the easy part is that you start back to back, not face to face. Know that being naked is a natural part of sexuality, and that your comfort level in your body will contribute to your erotic connection with your partner. The more comfortable you are in your body, the sexier you will feel.

You can do this exercise with the lights on or off. Try it first with the lights on low, or with candles lit. Make sure the room is warm enough so neither of you gets too cold to stand together naked. Make sure you have a comfortable floor to stand on.

Make sure the kids are taken care of and you have privacy.

Step One
Stand back to back with your partner, preferably naked. Notice what parts of your body are touching. See whether you can get more of your body parts to touch. Can you press tighter against each other? Is there a way to press up against each other's whole body?

Step Two

Now turn around without losing contact. Touch each other's body as much as possible as you slowly turn around.

Step Three

Now feel the front of your bodies touching. See whether you can get more of your body parts to touch. See whether you can press together and get your whole bodies to touch. Can you press tighter against each other? What other parts need to touch to add more togetherness? What parts feel the most alive?

Step Four

Tell each other exactly where you think your partner can move closer to you. Tell your partner where you like to feel him close to you. Ask your partner to rub against any parts of you where friction feels good. Close your eyes and feel the texture of each other's skin.

Step Five

Now separate slowly. Feel each body part leave the contact of your partner's body. Notice what the space feels like.

Step Six

Reconnect. Take your partner's hand and place it where you want more contact. Press his or her hand using all of yours—palm, fingers, the pads of your fingers— on that area. Connect with all of your hand. Feel the heat and energy from your partner's hand. Move your hand closer and make more contact.

Step Seven

Slowly remove your partner's hand and feel the disconnect.

Step Eight

Switch.

Step Nine

Continue moving your partner's hand over your body. Move your hands over your partner's body now. Feel the heat and energy coming off your partner's body. Notice which areas of her body are cool, warm, soft, or rough. Notice with curiosity and openness and without judgment the different private parts of the body and also the more public parts that show every day. See whether you can appreciate the parts in a new way, as if you are seeing them with your hands. Feel the passion and the energy rise.

Holding an Appreciation Night

In general, women need to feel emotionally connected before they have sex, and men feel emotionally connected after they have sex.

A couple can never share too many appreciations. This next exercise will help you to feel connected, and help women feel the emotional readiness to be open to sex.

EXERCISE

Appreciation Night

Make an appointment with your partner to hold an appreciation night at a time that works for both of you.

Remember in the previous appreciation exercises you learned to mirror back everything your partner says, without agreeing, refusing, explaining, or denying. Just be a "flat" mirror, which means to reflect back exactly what your partner says, no more and no less.

In this exercise we will also practice **summarizing** before we empathize and validate. The first receiver will summarize what he or she has heard.

Find a comfortable place to sit or lie down for at least fifty minutes. Make sure the kids are taken care of and you have total privacy. Create a sexy atmosphere by lighting candles or incense, putting on soft music, or having a sexy movie playing in the background.

Try to make eye contact with your partner, sitting close enough so that you can reach out and touch if it feels appropriate in the moment.

Know that this exercise may make you feel embarrassed, awkward, or silly. Take a deep breath when you feel this way. Notice how your pulse quickens and your heart races. Remember that this is part of the excitement of the exercise.

Step One

Decide who will be the sender and who will be the receiver. The sender will share the following three appreciations with his or her partner, one at a time:

- One thing you appreciated about your partner when you first met
- One thing you appreciate about your relationship now
- One thing you appreciate about sex with your partner

Step Two

After the sender sends over the first appreciation, the receiver mirrors back. It may sound like this:

Sender: "One thing I appreciated about you when I met you was how outspoken you were about your feelings for me."

Receiver (mirroring): "So one thing you really appreciated about me when you met me was how outspoken I was about my feelings for you."

Do this until you've sent over all three appreciations and had each one mirrored back.

Step Three

The receiver now summarizes all three appreciations.

Receiver: "So one thing you appreciated about me when we first met was how outspoken I was about my feelings for you, and one thing you appreciate about our relationship now is (for example) how attentive I am to your needs, and one thing you appreciate about sex with me is how I always make sure I give you an orgasm before I have one. Did I get that?"

Sender: "Yes" (or no, if the receiver has missed anything).

Step Four

The receiver validates what the sender has said.

Receiver: "It makes sense to me that you would appreciate those things, knowing you the way I know you, because of … . Did I get that?"

Sender: "Yes, you got that" (or add what the receiver might have missed).

Step Five

The receiver empathizes with the sender.

(continued on page 70)

(continued)

Receiver: "And I can imagine that having all those things makes you feel ..." (say any emotions that you think your partner may be experiencing).

Sender: "Yes, you got me."

Step Six

Switch.

Notice what happens when you are through with sharing this exercise. How are you feeling? Do you feel softer toward your partner? What are you feeling in your body? Do you feel any sexual stirrings or physical longings for your partner? Do you feel sexier? Turned on? Share with your partner what the exercise brought up for you.

Ravishment versus Rape

Over the past few decades, women have made great strides in working against sexual violence and abuse. The rape of women and the prevalence of violence and sex in the media, movies, rock videos, and society in general has led to a societal backlash of "no means no."

Feminists, lawmakers, police forces, and others have led the way to educate a male-driven society about the difference between sex and violence. Our laws now protect the victims of sexual violence and allow for broader representation, giving women a stronger voice and taking the violence out of sex.

In America we have feminized sex, which is a good thing, because it educated both men and women that rape is a violent act, not a sexual act. And yet, even though we've made progress, something has slipped through the cracks. Maybe we have confused sex for both men and women and mistakenly taken the passion out of sex.

For example, we have begun to teach men about the positive aspects of intimacy and sex. We have shown them how to touch our face, and be emotionally available and loving, which is wonderful! And yet women spend billions of dollars each year on bodice-ripping paperback novels, where some big, strong man throws the woman down on the bed and tears off her dress.

Maybe we have confused sex for both men and women and mistakenly taken the passion out of sex.

So what do women really want? Perhaps their desires include both tenderness and ravishment.

Being ravished means being swept off your feet, having your partner be crazy with love and desire for you, and being carried away by the moment. Being ravished can be a moment of pure and sublime bliss, because it allows for total surrender and trust.

Being ravished is a trust exercise, because it demands a ravisher and a ravishee. There must be a "yes" or permission from the one being ravished. This is what separates it from rape. And also what makes it hot and erotic. When the ravishee gives permission to be ravished, he or she is allowing someone else to take control, which allows the one being ravished to feel in control!

Letting go and having fun can mean acting out a sexual ravishment scene, as in the next exercise. This can be the beginning of role-playing and a way to experiment with the feeling of being vulnerable, and of being in control. Switching back and forth allows for both partners to experience the delight of how that can feel, and what it feels like to be the one letting go and being totally taken over by the desire of the other. And playing the role of the lover doing the ravishing can be a titillating experience of being in control and directing the other's pleasure.

Would you rather be ravished or be the ravisher in bed? Decide who will go first in this next exercise.

EXERCISE
Ravishment

Find a time where you and your partner will be free to act out your most erotic ravishment fantasy. Start with the idea that one of you will be totally in control, while the other will be totally naked (literally), and vulnerable to the erotic moment.

(continued on page 72)

(continued)

Set the mood by lighting candles, or by having a date night first. Come home and don't waste time. Start immediately, without waiting for permission. Remember, you have already gotten permission when you each decided who would be naked and who would be the ravisher. Now is the time to play!

Keep in mind that this is all in the spirit of erotic play and that you can laugh and giggle at any time. You don't have to keep up the role-play at all times. Experiment with how much you want to play the role, and take a breather if you have to.

If the ravishee at any time says "no," then stop and take a break. But remember to tell each other another word that might be fun to play with, like "stop," that the ravishee can say during the heat of the moment, but not really mean it.

This can add an element of danger that feels real, but is really playacting. (In a later exercise we will talk about safe words and why they are so important.)

Step One

Choose which partner will be naked tonight and which will be the ravisher. Those doing the ravishing will keep all of their clothes on. The ravisher can build up to taking the ravishee's clothes off slowly, torturing him or her with the exquisiteness of the subtle desire that is created by the waiting game. But remember, ravishment really means making the other person feel he or she is being taken over. Rough kissing, gentle hair pulling, stretching clothes, and yanking them off are fun ways to get into the make-believe of the ravishment fantasy.

Start any way you feel comfortable. Remember that the ravisher is in charge and will take off the ravishee's clothes in any way desired.

Step Two

When and if the ravishment turns into sex, the ravisher gets to decide whether to start slow or go fast and quick (remember, the ravishee has given permission for this to happen). Having sex with much of the ravisher's clothes on will keep the feeling of being in control paramount. Opening key clothing areas is, of course, permitted.

Know that next time, you will switch. But for this evening or afternoon, stay in the role until you are all the way through the exercise, or until you have had sex for the evening and can de-role.

Step Three

Afterward, talk about what it was like for you, and what you appreciated about being in the role of ravisher, and what you appreciated about being in the role of ravishee.

Reacting to Fantasies

Talking about our fantasies is risky business. For some, it might feel like sharing a private and intimate part of ourselves that we have never shared before. For others it might feel like something that we just don't talk about. And yet telling our partners about our most private thoughts is a way to feel connected and intimate with them.

Having the experience of being heard in a safe way by our partners is a way of helping them heal as well as a way to help us heal. The feeling of being held, being truly heard and listened to, and being seen for who we really are can heal us from the wounds of our past.

Many times, the one sharing the fantasies feels such a sense of gratitude and relief just for the opportunity to be heard that he begins to experience a new connection with his partner. True intimacy is achieved in those moments and remembered afterward.

Sometimes the telling of a fantasy alone is enough to create a heightened sense of erotic stimulation and connectedness within the sexual relationship.

Sometimes, as the receiver of this information, hearing about your partner's fantasies can be difficult. What if the fantasy involves something you are not comfortable with, or feel threatened by?

One way to deal with hearing a partner's fantasy that makes you uncomfortable is to simply mirror your partner. Just sitting with him allows your partner to express himself fully. Sometimes his fantasies are just fantasies, and he may never really want to take them into action. Perhaps he has wanted to tell these fantasies for a long time. Imagine how safe he would perceive you to be and how warm and loving he might feel toward you for simply listening to his fantasies.

When we first hear a fantasy, it can be a little surprising and sometimes create tension and uncertainty. We can feel unsure of whether our partner wants us to live out this fantasy, and sometimes unclear about where the fantasy comes from. Maybe it makes us wonder whether our partner has always wanted this, and perhaps has felt dissatisfied up until now. All these feelings are simply a story we make up based on our initial reaction to hearing the fantasy. With some time to digest, and hearing more about what our partner is thinking, it can become clearer to us, and we may begin to empathize.

It might make sense when we give ourselves the space to think about it, or to listen for more information, how our partner might want this. It might not make sense from our perspective, because perhaps we don't share the same fantasy. But this is what makes a relationship healthy and exciting. We are differentiated in our needs. What we want is many times different than what our partner wants. We don't have to be turned on or excited by the same things.

Learning to appreciate what our partner thinks and fantasizes about can be a key element in seeing our partner as sexy and alive.

EXERCISE
Sharing and Summing Up

Take some time together, perhaps on a date night, or create an evening where you have at least thirty minutes of uninterrupted time together, to review the exercises you have done so far in this book.

Spend some time talking to your partner about how the exercises have made you feel. Tell your partner what you have appreciated about him or her for doing the exercises with you, and talk about one thing you have learned about yourself from doing the exercises.

You may feel differently about your relationship now. Can you tell your partner? You might feel more anxious or a little scared that you have stretched into new areas. You may feel more excited and passionate toward your partner, and more excited about your relationship. You might also feel hope about the future of your relationship, honoring that there is an ongoing passionate connection available to you both, just by talking about your most intimate fantasies and appreciating each other.

Step One
Decide who will be the sender and who will be the receiver. The dialogue should start off like this:

Sender: "These exercises made me feel sexy."

Receiver (mirroring): "These exercises made you feel sexy."

Sender: "Particularly in the exercise about pressing our bodies together."

Receiver (mirroring): "So that particular exercise made you feel sexy."

Sender: "You got me."

Receiver (validating): "It makes sense that you would feel that because I know how much physical closeness means to you."

Sender: "You got me."

Receiver (empathizing): "I can imagine that doing those exercises also made you feel emotionally closer. Did I get that?"

Sender: "Yes, you got it."

Step Two
Switch.

Step Three
Follow the dialogue pattern in Step One, only the sender starts off with the following:

Sender: "One thing I learned about myself was (for example) that I really enjoy pleasing you."

Receiver (mirroring): "One thing you learned about yourself was that you really enjoy pleasing me."

Sender: "Particularly in the exercise about sharing our fantasies."

Receiver (mirroring): "So in that particular exercise you learned (for example) that you really enjoy pleasing me and that taught you something about yourself."

Sender: "You got me."

Receiver (validating): "It makes sense that you would feel you learned that because it sounds like you have learned that somtimes pleasing me makes you feel good too."

Sender: "You got me."

Receiver (empathizing): "I can imagine that learning that made you feel (for example) interested in learning more about yourself and finding out new ways to have better sex. Did I get that?"

Sender: "Yes, you got it."

Step Four
Switch.

(continued on page 76)

(continued)

Step Five

Follow the dialogue pattern in the above steps, only the sender starts off with the following:

Sender: "One thing I appreciated about you doing these exercises with me was how open you were with me."

The receiver then mirrors, validates, and empathizes with the sender.

Step Six

Switch.

Step Seven

Follow the dialogue pattern in the above steps, only the sender starts off with the following:

Sender: "One way I feel differently about our relationship is (for example) that I feel like I can tell you anything."

The receiver then mirrors, validates, and empathizes with the sender.

Step Eight

Switch.

The Payoff of Sexual Empathy: Passionate Closeness

4

Sexual empathy provides the safety and connection that allows for the exploration of fantasies. It means trying to understand how another person might want something different sexually than what we want.

Sexual empathy is also about perception. Do we know how empathetic our partner is? How understanding would they be if we were to tell them our most secret sexual fantasy—do we know or are we just guessing? And are you, as a partner, sexually empathic? Does your partner perceive you as someone willing to explore his or her sexual fantasies?

The payoff in being sexually empathic is huge. The power in the relationship is always held by the one with the most sexual empathy. Being the partner who can be open and understanding regardless of the topic means that you are perceived by your partner as being open enough in the relationship to talk about anything. If your partner knows he can tell you anything, then passion doesn't need to get split off outside the safe confines of the relationship.

Sexual empathy leads to improved communication and sexual generosity. When we know our partner can hear us, listen to us, and not judge our deepest fantasies and desires, there is a greater likelihood that these desires will become a reality.

Working together to increase sexual empathy prevents the need to go outside of the relationship to get your sexual needs met. It channels the erotic energy *into* the relationship. This increases the energy and loving feelings between partners, and it improves communication, sexual safety, and respect in the relationship.

The power in the relationship is always held by the one with the most sexual empathy.

When Empathy Is Lacking

Let's take two scenarios based on what could happen with and without sexual empathy in a relationship. Average husband and typical wife go to a couple's therapy session. They are encouraged to communicate with each other about their sexual needs. Average husband tells his wife he has a fantasy he would like to share with her. A low sexually empathetic response would be something like this.

Average husband: "Honey, I have a fantasy of seeing you dressed in sexy lingerie and waiting for me when I get home from work."

Typical wife: "Oh sure, like I have nothing better to do."

After a conversation like this, where one partner uses sarcasm, the partner who took the risk in sharing his or her fantasy will feel misunderstood and put off. We use sarcasm and defensiveness with our partner because we don't know how to empathize. Because of our own feelings, we might find it hard to respond to our partner's desires with understanding and compassion. We can't put ourselves in our partner's shoes, because we resist trying to understand his feelings.

Even if it doesn't make any sense to us that our partner wants to see us dressed up, it might make perfect sense to us that he might want that. If we can understand where he is coming from, we have an opportunity to be empathetic and show we care about his feelings and desires.

How Imago Can Help

Using the Imago dialogue, we can get past some of our resistance, and instead of deflecting our partner's requests and desires, we can respond in a way that feels empathic and understanding. When our partner feels our empathy, even if we don't agree to do anything, there is room for more satisfying sexual possibilities.

With the Imago dialogue, showing empathy starts by mirroring what our partner has said, which gives us a caring and respectful way to respond to our partner when he expresses a fantasy. Many times, having the structure of the dialogue helps us to hold our "reactivity" when we hear something that surprises us, or something that we don't understand.

"Reactivity" is the behavior, such as sarcasm or distancing, that shows up in our relationships when we react to our partners in a way that may hurt their feelings. Our reactivity is a response to something that hurts or angers us. If we don't take a moment to try and understand where our partners are coming from, we are more likely to go into a reactive and defensive mode. When we pull away from our partners, it can feel like we are doing it to protect ourselves from hurt, yet they will perceive it as abandonment or rejection. If we attack our partners when we are afraid or angry, then our partners will feel intruded upon, and they may become reactive in response.

This creates an unhealthy cycle of pursue and withdraw. When one person withdraws and the other pursues, no one is really making a connection. And we probably aren't getting the sex we want!

What Sexual Empathy Sounds Like

Giving a sexually empathic response to our partners when they share a fantasy means only that we mirror back what they have said. This gives time to think about what they are asking before there is a need for a response. It also allows us to really take the time to listen to their fantasy.

This feels much safer to our partners than when we attack them or withdraw from the relationship. Sharing a fantasy can make our partners feel vulnerable and exposed, and this can be a big risk. If we can help our partners feel safe while exposing their most private and intimate thoughts and desires, they will see us as a caring and empathic lover.

A sexually empathic response might sound like this:

Average husband: "Honey, I have a fantasy of seeing you dressed in sexy lingerie and waiting for me when I get home from work."

Typical wife: "So, okay, let me see if I got this … you have a fantasy of seeing me dressed in sexy lingerie and waiting for you when you get home from work?"

In a sexually empathic relationship, all we have to do is mirror back what is being said using the Imago techniques. As stated above, this response gives us time to think about what our partner is saying and time to react. We don't have to rush into action before we are ready. There is time to decide about acting out the fantasy later. Right now, having the dialogue about sex is the most important thing, as it will increase the sexual empathy in the relationship, allowing for the development of trust and safety.

As this ongoing trust is created in your relationship, a new type of energy may emerge between you. Feeling safe and open with your partner can be the beginning of a new type of erotic connection. Your ability to be verbal about sex and share with your partner your deepest desires and fantasies creates a space that allows for further experimentation and risk. Risk can't happen unless you trust your partner to receive your efforts with empathy and understanding. Your partner will in turn be more likely to move to an action phase, helping you move your fantasies into reality.

EXERCISE
Exploring Sexual Empathy

This exercise will build on the dialogue skills you learned in the earlier chapters and incorporate more validation and empathy.

For this exercise, you are adding new and exciting elements to your dialogue and telling your partner what you want to do to him or her. By now you have a new form of communication, the Imago dialogue. All your partner has to do is listen, using the Imago dialogue skills. He or she can listen actively by mirroring, validating, and empathizing. This type of empathic conversation creates a safe structure in which to talk about your erotic thoughts and fantasies.

Using the Imago dialogue, tell your partner the following:

- What you always wanted to try sexually

- One thing you would like to do for your partner sexually

- One thing you would like to do sexually while your partner watches

These statements might feel a little riskier than in earlier dialogues. Doing the sexual empathy exercise will make you aware of how to talk about and risk sharing your true feelings and desires. So take some risks! Do the exercise and use some of the sexy language you have practiced in previous exercises.

For this first exercise, you will need at least forty-five minutes of uninterrupted private time with your partner. Find a quiet place where you can talk comfortably, either sitting up or lying down together. Make sure you face each other and make eye contact when you share this dialogue with each other.

As in the previous exercises, we will be sharing and then mirroring. Although you may have practiced these dialogue skills already, you might still feel uncomfortable with the slow pace that this creates in your "conversation." See if you can appreciate the slower pace of the dialogue and notice how it brings you closer to your partner, allowing you to appreciate each word and nuance of emotion in what he or she is saying to you.

In addition, you will be validating and empathizing with your partner, adding a new level of understanding and safety to the conversation. You may have to stretch to mirror and validate your partner's desires, and with practice, the more difficult language will become more comfortable. Soon you will have a safe way to talk to your partner about your fears. This is a great place to create the empathic relationship you will need later on as you take more risks together.

Step One

First, choose who will be the sender and who will be the receiver. As stated above, senders will tell their partner the following:

- What you always wanted to try sexually

The receiver will simply repeat, or mirror, what the sender says. It is important in an empathic dialogue that you don't add any of your own reactivity, and mirror exactly what your partner sends over.

An example might be the following:

Sender: "What I have always wanted to try is to have sex together in the shower."

The receiver simply mirrors back, maintaining eye contact, "So, what you have always wanted to try is to have sex together in the shower."

There are only two responses receivers need to make at this point—either "please send that again" or "Is there more?" The sender can say "yes" and send more or "no" and stop there.

(continued on page 82)

(continued)

Step Two

Senders then say, for example, "One thing I would like to do for you sexually is give you a back rub." Receivers mirror back what the senders said.

Step Three

Senders then say, for example, "One thing I would like to do sexually while you watch is masturbate." Receivers mirror back what the senders said.

Step Four

After the sender has sent all three desires and the receiver has mirrored them back, the receiver summarizes all of them by saying, "So what I heard you say was … ."

Step Five

The receiver then validates each statement, starting with, "It makes sense to me you would want to try … knowing you the way I know you, I can understand why you would desire that." This format makes validation easier.

Step Six

Now empathize, which means to guess at what you think your partner would feel if she had these desires and fantasies fulfilled. For example:

Receiver: "And I can imagine that if you did those things it would make you feel … (add feelings). Is there more?"

Step Seven

Now switch and your partner will have a turn to summarize, validate, and empathize.

If now is not a good time, or if further dialogue is needed to find empathy, then ask for another time to talk further about your desires and fantasies. Making a plan to keep talking until you feel openness and trust in the relationship. There is no rush. Just hearing about each other's sexual and erotic desires might add enough spark and excitement that making love spontaneously is definitely a possibility!

What Prevents Sexual Empathy?

Sometimes we want to be sexually empathic and, for whatever reason, cannot. One reason this happens is that our own personal fears and anxieties keep us from being sexually empathic toward our partner. If we feel shame about our own curiosity, it becomes difficult to be empathic with our partner.

We all fear being judged. Our inner fantasy life is often so personal and many times so secret that just the thought of sharing these feelings with another person can create anxiety and shame.

We are ultimately afraid that we will lose our connection with our partner over our deepest sexual needs. We may have a desire to tone down our thoughts and fantasies because we don't want to hurt the other person.

And finally, we use something called "projection" to justify how we think the other person will feel and react to us if we share our sexual fantasies. We project how we feel onto our partners: "If I feel this way, then so will he. If I think that certain sexual acts and desires are 'weird,' then so will my partner." Most times, in actuality, we have no idea how our partners will react, even when we have known them for a long time.

Sexual Empathy Contributes to Long-Term Happiness

Couples with a higher level of sexual empathy have a greater likelihood of staying together in the long term because they are more satisfied. Increasing sexual empathy in the relationship develops deeper connections. Sexually empathetic couples process and communicate their fantasies in healthy, relaxed ways and consequently maintain lasting satisfaction in their relationships.

Couples who identify what they are erotically curious about increase the feeling of sexual empathy in their partnership. They learn to normalize their curiosity and fantasies and can communicate with each other about their desires.

When couples explore their erotic curiosity with each other, sharing their fantasies safely, they can learn how to make all of their dreams come true and really have the sex they want.

Sexually empathetic couples process and communicate their fantasies in healthy, relaxed ways and consequently maintain lasting satisfaction in their relationships.

Our erotic needs include a desire for safety and trust, but also a craving for deep connection and intensity. Some levels of "safety" in a relationship may feel like boredom or being stuck. This is different than being in a sexually empathetic relationship, where it is safe to share feelings about sex.

Communication exercises where couples can learn to ask for their erotic needs to be met and explore fantasies together help solidify the freedom in a relationship. The capacity to tolerate and talk about the anxiety that hearing another's fantasy might bring up makes a relationship stronger.

How to talk, touch, and improve the sex and sensuality in a relationship, and being present for the other, are the goals of the erotic partnership.

When we learn how to be authentic with each other, we find a renewed intimacy in our relationship.

Taking More Risks

This next exercise will flex your fantasy muscles. You are now getting more comfortable talking to your partner about sex. Now you have a structure in which to ask for specific things you like. Now you can begin to get in touch with your own inner fantasy life.

Educating your partner about your fantasy life is the only way to give your partner the opportunity to give you what you want. You are teaching your partner how to love you. Give your partner the tools to do that, and he will feel more successful at it, and you will feel like you are getting the sex you want.

Flex Your Fantasy Muscles

For this exercise, you will explore your own internal fantasy world first, and then share these thoughts with your partner. You will need a quiet place to sit down and write, along with a pen and paper or a journal. Take about thirty minutes of uninterrupted quiet time to think and describe in detail your thoughts.

You will need another sixty minutes of quiet private time with your partner to dialogue about what you have written. These two parts of the exercise can be done at two separate times or at the same time. You might want to have this dialogue on a date night, when you can concentrate on each other and listen to each other's inner fantasies.

Step One

First, get out your paper or journal, and answer the following questions. Try to include as much detail as you can, such as where you would be, what you would wear, what your partner would be doing, and so on.

- Write down one sexual thing in bed that you love to do.

- Write down one sexual thing that your partner might want to do.

- Write down one sexual fantasy you have that you haven't told your partner.

Step Two

Now ask for the time to share with your partner what you have written. Find a comfortable place to sit or lie down where you can make eye contact with your partner as you share what you have written about your fantasies.

Senders "send" over their desires in their first statement. Receivers simply repeat, or mirror, what the sender says. Take turns going through each step, sending and mirroring. It is important in an empathetic dialogue that you don't add any of your own reactivity, and simply mirror exactly what your partner says.

An example might be the following:

Sender: "One sexual thing that I love to do in bed is to be on top."

The receiver simply mirrors back, maintaining eye contact:

Receiver: "So, one thing that you love to do in bed is to be on top."

After the receiver has mirrored, the sender switches and becomes the receiver.

(continued on page 86)

(continued)

Step Three

After you've both shared and mirrored, summarize what each other has said. Receiver: "So what I heard you say was (summarize all three desires)." Ask your partner to remind you if you've forgotten part of what he or she said.

Step Four

Next, validate what each other has said. Using the sentence frame "It makes sense to me …" makes this easier. How does it make sense to you, knowing your partner the way you do, that he or she would like these things and want to do more of them with you?

Step Five

Next, empathize with what your partner has said. Remember, it might be a stretch to do this, but you are an empathic partner now and you can listen in this active way. You don't ever have to commit to living out your partner's fantasies until you are comfortable.

Receiver: "And I can imagine that if you did those things it would make you feel (add feelings). Is there more?"

Step Six

Now switch and your partner will have a turn to summarize, validate, and empathize.

You can move on from here if you are both comfortable, and each of you can choose one thing your partner has expressed a desire for. Remember that you are giving your partner a gift of living out a fantasy. This generosity comes from the sexual empathy you now have for your partner, a deeper understanding of his or her thoughts, feelings, and desires.

If now is not a good time, then ask for another time to talk more about your desires and fantasies. Making a plan to keep talking until your partner understands you can create openness in the relationship. Just hearing about your sexual and erotic desires might add enough spark and excitement that making love spontaneously is definitely a possibility!

Bridging the Sexual Communication Gap 5

Taking erotic communication to the next step, we can use the Imago techniques we have learned so far to help bridge the separation that sometimes exists in sexual partnerships.

Men and women have different communication styles, and within a relationship partners have differing comfort levels talking about sex. How honest we are with each other about our sexual needs is dependent on what we have learned about sex and our bodies, as well as the rules and customs with which we grew up. It is also contingent on how much we trust our partner to listen and validate our desires.

In our society, there is a lot of confusion when it comes to sexuality and sexual relationships. This confusion makes it difficult for us to identify our sexual needs and even harder to talk about them. We are unsure about how to ask for what we want sexually, what words to use, and what is acceptable for discussion.

Being honest with ourselves about our desires is not as clear-cut as it may appear at first glance. If we were honest with ourselves about what we craved, then we could be honest with our partner about our desires. However, many times we aren't sure.

Being sexually honest with our partner means taking the risk to share what is going on in our bodies. It means telling our partner what feels good and what might feel better. It means having a language to describe what may not be working and what would work better. It means having an open dialogue and a level of comfort with each other to talk about our sexual needs. This can help us get the sex we want, and it can help us give our partner what he or she really wants in bed.

Unfortunately, figuring out what our partner wants in bed can sometimes feel like adolescent fumbling in the back seat of a car. We stumble around our partner's body until we hit on something that seems to work, and many times we repeat that same move and style every time we make love, because we have found the "right button to push." If our partners want something different or want to try sex a different way, it can be hard for them to be honest with us without worrying that they will hurt our feelings.

EXERCISE
Sexual Honesty Questionnaire

Use the questionnaire below to gauge you and your partner's sexual honesty.

Answer the questions below, using a scale from 1 to 5, with 1 meaning never/not at all and 5 meaning always/very much so.

Rate your answers to your questions and share them with your partner. There is no right or wrong way to do this exercise, so answer quickly and without judgment.

1	2	3	4	5
Never	Sometimes	Many times	Usually	Always

I talk freely about sex with my partner.

1   2   3   4   5

I think it is important to our relationship to be intimate.

1   2   3   4   5

I am satisfied with our sex life.

1   2   3   4   5

There are things I would like to try if my partner was open to the idea.

1   2   3   4   5

I have thoughts and fantasies about new things to do in bed.

1   2   3   4   5

I am confident I can ask for what I fantasize about.

1   2   3   4   5

I feel good about my body.

1   2   3   4   5

I would like help from my partner to indicate where he/she likes to be touched.

1   2   3   4   5

I would like help from my partner to indicate where her clitoris is located.

1   2   3   4   5

I would like help from my partner to indicate where her G-spot is located.

1   2   3   4   5

My partner and I talk freely about any sexual dysfunction in our relationship, for example, premature ejaculation, difficulty in maintaining or achieving erection, or not ejaculating.

1   2   3   4   5

My partner can achieve orgasm through clitoral stimulation.

1   2   3   4   5

My partner can achieve orgasm through vaginal stimulation.

1   2   3   4   5

My partner can achieve orgasm through vaginal and clitoral stimulation.

1   2   3   4   5

I would like assistance from my partner to locate spots along the vaginal wall and the outside labia that feel good when stimulated.

1   2   3   4   5

I know what the perineum is and where it is located on my partner.

1   2   3   4   5

(continued on page 90)

(continued)

I know what the male prostate gland is and how it is stimulated in my partner.

1   2   3   4   5

I am open to anal stimulation from my partner.

1   2   3   4   5

I would like to experience anal sex, either for the first time or more often.

1   2   3   4   5

I would like help from my partner to indicate how she would like her clitoris stimulated.

1   2   3   4   5

I would like help from my partner to indicate how she would like her vagina stimulated.

1   2   3   4   5

I would like help from my partner to indicate specifically the ways in which he enjoys having his penis stimulated.

1   2   3   4   5

I know where my partner's scrotum is located.

1   2   3   4   5

My partner enjoys having his scrotum stimulated.

1   2   3   4   5

I would like help from my partner to indicate how he would like his scrotum stimulated.

1   2   3   4   5

I have a sincere desire to talk more openly with my partner about our sex life.

1   2   3   4   5

Add up your score. If you have a lot of 4s and 5s, you are more open and ready to be sexually honest with your partner. If you have more 1s and 2s you are ready to work on opening up to your partner in safer and healthier ways.

Types of Arousal

Many times our partner's erotic fantasy life is different from our own because their body is different, as are their arousal levels and points of intensity.

Arousal levels differ among women, too, depending on their sensitivity, hormone levels, and psychological openness to the experience of sexuality. Men have differing levels of arousal depending on age, mood, and energy level.

We also vary as people depending on what stimulus creates arousal in our bodies. Some of us are visual, with a high level of turn-on based on seeing things like our partner's naked body. Some of us are tactile, which means that touch, of a varying sort, can arouse us to stimulation. Some people are aural, meaning they get aroused hearing sounds and words.

Figuring out what our arousal points are and learning about our partner's are part of the wonderful erotic discovery possible through communication.

Ask whether your partner is more visual, tactile, or aural during sex. Help your partner identify which area is the most intense. You might think you know what turns your partner on. And you may be right, but now is your chance to find out.

EXERCISE
Your Partner's Senses

This exercise can be the beginning of the sexual honesty that leads to long-term passion. Learning to be honest with each other is key. Sexual honesty is about engaging our partners in conversation about what turns them on.

First, find a time that will allow you enough uninterrupted privacy that you and your partner will feel comfortable exploring each other's senses. Warm up the room by raising the heat, lowering the lights, and creating an atmosphere of sensual discovery. Make sure you set up things in the room that your partner can see and smell, such as fresh flowers. Add something sensual your partner can hear, like jazz, classical music, or light rock. And also add something in the room that feels wonderful against the skin, such as silk sheets or soft pillows.

(continued on page 92)

(continued)

You will also need some props for this exercise. Find a soft feather or clean feather duster, an ice cube, a hairbrush, and anything else you think might feel sensual against your partner's skin. Find a blindfold or a silk scarf.

Step One

Decide who will be the sender and who will be the receiver. Receivers should lie comfortably on the bed and remove as much clothing as they are comfortable with. Senders should ask receivers whether it is okay to tie the blindfold over their eyes. Then get comfortable, and dazzle your partner with sensual delights.

Step Two

Focus on your partner's sense of hearing by whispering in his ear. Whisper the things you are planning to do to his tactile senses, through the skin. This might sound like:

"I am going to gently touch your skin ... ."

Then take the feather and lightly tickle and brush the skin with it.

Take the ice cube and slide it over his warm body until it melts.

Then take the brush and very gently scratch your partner with the bristles.

The idea is to give him a heightened tactile experience, while whispering in his ear for his aural pleasure.

Step Three

Now slowly take off the blindfold and let him see what you are doing to him. This will add visual stimulation.

Step Four

Now ask him what he liked the most. "Do you like when I talk to you? Do you like when I touch you? Do you like to watch me touch you? Tell me what you like the most ... ."

If you want to keep going and make love at this point, save the "switch" part of this exercise for next time.

Step Five

Switch.

Navigating Arousal

Helping your partner learn the "arousal map" of your body is important to sexual connection. An "arousal map" contains the patterns and sensitivity in your body that are unique to your physical self. Your partner has his or her own arousal map, too.

No one gives us a map to each other's body when we meet and fall in love. Part of the joy of an erotic relationship is exploring this landscape together. Without directions, we can wander joyfully and find places we like, yet still risk missing some of the more important and delightful places on our lover's body. With interaction, we can go back and forth together, exploring, learning, and growing as a sexual couple.

What Sex Ed Didn't Tell Us

Growing up, we learn in health education classes about the egg and the sperm, but we don't receive the "manual" for the opposite sex's body. As young people, we can be confused about how the opposite sex feels in his or her body. We might know how the internal organs work from health class or anatomy, but we don't learn about how the opposite sex reaches arousal levels or orgasm. This is something we fumble with later on as we grow into relationships.

As adolescents and adults, our confusion about our partner's body might be resolved subtly over time, as we explore and delight in each other's differences. (Same-sex couples have this experience as well. Exploring another person's body is intriguing, even if it has the same parts as ours—because the other person still has differences in arousal points and levels.) But most of us are still unsure about how to fully engage our partners sexually, unless they tell us how.

Growing up, we are not only confused about the opposite sex but also about our own growing bodies and newly developing sexual desires. When we mature and engage in erotic relationships, we begin to discover our sexuality, and if we learn to be sexually honest with our partners, we give them a way to bring us the pleasure we desire, and we open a dialogue to learn to express our own needs, learning more about ourselves in the process.

Learning how to talk about sex can be a hit-or-miss process. We might find a book or helpful partner to encourage us, but there is not a lot of information or training available to learn how to talk about sex with our partners. Lots of books discuss sexuality, but not how to talk about it with the people we are having sex with.

Our culture does not make it easy to talk about sex. We can see sex in the media, in magazines, and in the movies, but no one seems to be able to talk about it openly and honestly.

The Imago dialogue process of mirroring and validation can help bridge this gap and also any differences in our communication styles. Sometimes it's hard to verbalize our needs, and having someone listen in this empathetic way can make it easier to say what may feel awkward or uncomfortable. Listening to our partner use these dialogue skills gives us a new level of mastery over sexual communication.

How Other Cultures Approach Sexual Education

In some cultures, boys are initiated into sexuality by an older, more experienced woman, who shares the ways of eroticism with them so that they may pass it on to less experienced girls.

In other cultures, boys are introduced to sex in brothels and by prostitutes, paid for by their families. In today's age of AIDS and other sexually transmitted diseases, these practices may be less common than in the past. Many cultures are now similar to ours, in that young people fumble and grope as an introduction to sexuality, where once the elders of the society may have been more involved and supportive in the sexual development of their youth.

A Pattern of Dysfunction

If our relationships are complicated, then talking about sex can be the same as talking about anything else in a relationship—difficult. Whatever dysfunctional style of communication we have adapted in our partnership will most assuredly be acted out when we talk about our sexual needs.

Talking about sex can sometimes wound at a deeper level than other discussions. Because most people have some kind of insecurity around sexuality and performance, talking about sex with your partner can be a sensitive and difficult challenge. There is a risk of hurting each other's feelings, bruising egos, and using sarcasm or defensiveness to prevent open and honest sharing. We might not mean for this to happen, but we can get stuck in a pattern of relating to each other that makes it hard to reach a new level of openness. Many couples don't know where to begin to talk about sex honestly and with a level of vulnerability that helps them feel connected and intimate.

Whatever dysfunctional style of communication we have adapted in our partnership will most assuredly be acted out when we talk about our sexual needs.

Here is an example of what can happen when couples try to talk about sex. Sometimes other issues get dragged into the discussion along with sex.

Pete and Pam were not happy with their sex life. They began to talk about sex together one night after a long day fighting about money. Instead of using the Imago dialogue as a guide, they got into their regular pattern of relating to each other.

This pattern had been established long ago in their relationship. Pam had a long-standing resentment against Pete because she felt that he didn't understand that she needed to invest money in her business. She saw spending money as a necessity for the growth and expansion of their family. Pete saw Pam's spending as unnecessary. He felt that she should not invest any of their hard-earned capital in her business until it was established.

Pam took Pete's withholding financial support as being emotionally withholding. She felt this was a sign that he did not believe in her. Pete felt Pam disregarded his feelings about money and saw this as a lack of respect for him. Neither Pam nor Pete had insight into his or her own issues around money and spending, nor did they explore their deeper needs for acceptance and love, which were left over from their childhoods.

They both craved a deeper sexual connection, which would comfort them and make them feel more connected. Particularly after fighting about money, they both wanted an erotic experience that would make them feel more intimate with each other. For example, Pete wanted to share his fantasies with Pam.

One night, they thought that talking about sex might get them through their resentments that had been building all week. Pam asked Pete to talk about what he might be interested in trying. Finally he shared, cautiously at first. He told Pam, "I would like you to dress up in leather clothes during sex."

Pam immediately responded by saying, "Well, that's not going to happen because you wouldn't let me spend the money on leather clothes!"

Pete immediately shut down.

A Different Way of Sharing

If Pam and Pete had used the Imago dialogue and been able to mirror their fantasies, they could have slowed down this process, allowing time for receptivity and not reactivity. They could have experienced their conversation very differently. The Imago dialogue can hold a space that can be experienced by both as being generous and supportive.

Another way that conversation could have gone would be:

Pete: "Is now a good time to have a dialogue?"

Pam: "Yes."

Pete: "Is now a good time to talk about sex?"

Pam: "Yes, okay."

Pete: "I have a fantasy I would like to share with you."

Pam: "You have a fantasy you would like to share with me."

Pete: "One thing I really appreciate about you is the way you look in clothes."

Pam: "One think you really appreciate about me is the way I look in clothes."

Pete: "And one thing I have fantasized about but never shared is to see you dressed up in leather clothes."

Pam: "And one thing you have fantasized about but never shared is to see me dressed up in leather clothes. Is there more?"

Pete: "Yes, and specifically to have sex with you while you are wearing a leather thong."

Pam: "So specifically you have thought about having sex with me while I am wearing a leather thong. Is there more?"

Pete: "Just that it would mean a lot to me because I know this would be a stretch for you."

Pam: "So this would mean a lot to you because you know it would be a stretch for me. Is there more?"

Pete: "No, that's it."

Pam (validating): "Knowing you the way I know you, Pete, I understand you like to see me dressed up; you have always liked that. So it makes sense to me that you would want to see me in leather. And I know you like thongs, and would appreciate it if I stretched for you, since that is really not my thing. I can imagine that you would really appreciate it if I wore that for you."

Pete: "You got it!"

Pam (empathizing): "And I can imagine that if you got those things, if I were to wear leather and a leather thong while we had sex, that you would feel really turned on, and very loved, since it would be a stretch for me, and you would know I would be doing this just for you."

Pete: "Yes, it would be very sexy."

Pam: "So for you it would be very sexy."

Pete: "Yes."

Pam: "Did I get all your feelings?"

Pete: "I would also feel grateful."

Pam: "Oh, okay, and grateful."

Pete: "Yes, you got me!"

Pam, you'll notice, does not commit to acting out Pete's fantasy, nor does she judge him. She mirrors him, validates, and empathizes. This allows Pete to express his feelings honestly, and allows Pam time to absorb what he is asking. She can decide at another time whether she will actually take him up on his request.

She might think about it for a while, or fantasize about it herself, or even talk to him about it again at a later time. She could even talk to her girl-friends about it.

The Differences in Dialogue

Men are intrigued by women's conversations. Men want to understand not only how women's minds work, but also what they share with each other when men are not around. More important, men want to know what women actually say to each other about sex. Do they share details? Do they compare notes? Do they compare *them*?

Most men are amazed to hear that women talk about sex more often than men do, and with much more detail. Women, in groups, have a tendency to talk much more graphically about sexuality than men. Men, when in groups, often talk about women objectively and in generalized terms.

"Oh, yeah, last night was great, we had great sex ... ."

Or they look at women in the bar and comment, "Look at the breasts on her."

Women, while in groups, also objectify men, but they share intimate details of their own sexual scenarios. Women talk graphically about what happens in bed. For instance, a woman might explain what a man did to her sexually, describing her own multiorgasmic experience, but not necessarily detailing the man's performance.

The drive women have to share their feelings about relationships stems from both their history and their natural approach to problem solving. For example, women have spent eternity in community. Joined in the ancient, sacred bonding ritual of womanly sensual arts, women throughout the ages have gathered in red tents, in quilting bees, around the hearth, and at summer camps. During sleepovers, around the kitchen table, around the birthing bed, women have shared intimate details of their sex lives, opened up about their feelings, and talked about their relationships.

Women's natural tendency to express their emotions is part of their capacity for problem solving. Women talk until they have diluted the emotion attached to a problem. Men have a tendency to problem solve by finding solutions to problems, and therefore find women's capacity to repeatedly talk about a problem confusing and redundant.

EXERCISE
Learning the Language of Arousal

Learning how to communicate with your partner about the arousal levels in your body begins with identifying your own arousal patterns. You'll need a language to communicate this to your partner. Finally you also need a way for your partner to understand and translate what you are saying.

In this exercise, your partner will help you find the parts of your body that trigger the greatest levels of arousal, and will help you pinpoint the areas where you like the most concentrated touch. Your partner will also help you figure out what type of touch you like the most in those areas. How wonderful that you have someone to share this information with! Remember to appreciate your partner for his or her willingness to go on this exploratory journey with you.

(continued on page 100)

(continued)

For this exercise you will need at least sixty minutes of uninterrupted time. Make sure the children are taken care of and that your phone is turned off. Make sure the room you are using is quiet enough to be able to hear each other speak in a low tone of voice. Set the atmosphere by lighting candles, putting on soft background music, and making the bed with soft or silky sheets.

You can do this exercise with sexy and comfortable clothes on, or you can be naked, either taking turns or both of you disrobing before you begin.

In this exercise, your partner will touch you and you will respond verbally, using a number system to specifically identify how sensitive each section of your body surface feels. Numbers 1 to 10 will reflect how something feels as your partner touches you, with 1 meaning there is hardly any sensation and 10 meaning that the arousal and sensitivity level is at its peak.

Step One

Decide who will be the sender and who will be the receiver, and remember you get to switch, so you will each have a turn. Receivers will be the first to be touched and to express their reaction to each touch. You will use the number system to have a language to accurately describe the sensations and to give your partner clear information about the sensitive arousal map of your body.

Receivers should lie down in a comfortable position that they can sustain for at least thirty minutes. Senders should find a comfortable place to sit or lie with their prone partner, where they can reach all parts of their partner's body with little effort.

Step Two

First, receivers should tell their partners how much they appreciate them for doing this exercise with them. It might sound like: "I really appreciate you helping me find the sensitive areas of my body and helping me find a way to express that information to you."

Your partner, the sender, can mirror this back. "So you really appreciate that I am helping you find the sensitive areas of your body and helping you express that information to me."

Step Three

Now ask your partner to help you find the parts of your body that are most sensitive to touch. The sender now gently touches each area of the receiver's body, choosing small or large areas and caressing each spot until the receiver identifies a number of sensitivity.

Start on the outer parts of the body, furthest from the center of the torso. For example, starting with the hands or feet and moving inward will increase the arousal and sensitivity for the receiver as the touch gets closer to the more sensitive genital and nipple areas.

Receivers should relax, close their eyes, and feel each touch and caress. As the sender gently touches and caresses every part of the receiver's body, the receiver responds with a number from 1 to 10 to show how sensitive that area is. For example, the sender may touch the receiver's ankle. The receiver relaxes into the touch and decides how sensitive the area is, with 1 being little sensitivity and 10 being highly stimulated and aroused.

After being touched, the receiver might say, "That's a 4."

The sender then mirrors back, "So this is a 4."

Then the sender moves on to another area of the receiver's body.

The sender may want to try adjusting the touch and intensity of the caress. Perhaps the light touch on the receiver's ankle is a 4, and then the sender deepens the stroke and makes it a more massaging caress, and the receiver now shares that this feels like a 6. The sender mirrors back this information.

After varying the intensity of the strokes, from tender and gentle to firm and assured, vary the speed. Most people do not like simple repetitive movements over the same area for a long period of time. This can feel irritating.

Notice what speed or variety works the best to increase the level of sensitivity.

Notice that as you progress from the outer parts of the body to the inner parts of the body (closer to the center of the body) that the sensitivity level may increase.

Step Four

Now try to identify specific feelings associated with being touched on certain areas of your body. The sender should touch you gently or firmly in different areas. Senders should try to remember what the receivers responded to in the first part of the exercise. Did they feel more sensitive with a lighter stroke or a firmer caress?

The receiver can now say an adjective or descriptive word describing how it feels to be touched in each area. For example, if the sender touches the receiver's knee, the receiver could identify a feeling or reaction, such as, "That feels nice and soft."

The sender mirrors: "So that feels nice and soft."

(continued on page 102)

(continued)

If the sender touches a genital area, or more sensitive skin, the receiver might say, "That feels wonderful."

The sender then mirrors, "That feels wonderful."

Senders might try to think up words beforehand so that they have some in mind when the receiver begins to touch them.

Step Five

When you are through with each part of your partner's body, front and back, then switch.

(Another variation on this exercise: Combine this exercise with another. The receivers should be totally naked while the senders remained clothed. Receivers take turns identifying their levels of sensitivity by number, and then use feeling words as the sender touches different areas of their body. Save the "switch" for another night.)

If this exercise leads to lovemaking or erotic connection, great. If not, that's okay, too. Know that you have just discovered a huge amount of valuable information about your partner's arousal and her body's map of sensitive areas. You can use this information next time you make love or anytime you need a language to describe your body's response.

Step Six

Talk about any feelings that came up for both of you, and how it felt to do this exercise.

Step Seven

End with an appreciation for each other, both as the sender and as the receiver.

This exercise is a great way to work through some of the inherent shame attached to expressing and communicating sexual responsiveness. It also allows for a deeper level of intimacy and connection with your partner. Intimacy is a great aphrodisiac, and it can help keep the passionate part of your relationship alive for years to come.

Behind a Curtain of Shame:
Erotic Art History

We are all affected by our culture's view of sexuality, and we integrate this into our sex lives. Erotic connection is a normal and healthy part of a love relationship, and yet it is the most private and intimate part of connection.

A woman came into my office recently suffering from a feeling of distance in her relationship. She wanted to be closer to her partner, but was afraid to tell him how she felt and what she needed, and this made her feel sexually and emotionally distant from him.

On a recent business trip to New Mexico, she discovered that she came by this fear naturally, and that it was prevalent throughout our society and not just in her relationship. She learned from the experience and was able to take this trip home with her, "pulling her own curtains aside," and be more honest and open about her sexuality with her partner.

She told me the following story:

"I was in Taos recently, and wandering along the plaza, I stumbled on the La Fonda Hotel, hidden behind old green wooden doors since 1820. Wandering in out of the dust and hot sun, I found a small white sign that said 'D.H. Lawrence Forbidden Paintings, $3.'

"I crept further into the dark lobby, where a woman sat behind glass where there was a small opening at the bottom of her window hollowed out for sliding in money. I felt like I was at a peep show. I paid my $3 and the woman came out from behind the glass and led me into a back room.

"I was the only patron there to see the show, despite it being the peak of tourist season. I felt like I was about to enter into the secret world. (D.H. Lawrence was the author of *Lady Chatterley's Lover*, a drastically erotic novel for its day, published in 1928.) I wanted to be alone to see his paintings, but it was obvious that the guide was not going to leave me alone with the exhibit. She stood next to me and handed me a small piece of paper describing the paintings.

(continued on page 104)

Behind a Curtain (continued)

"She then told me to turn and face a large wall in this otherwise nondescript room filled with dining tables and a podium. She slowly pulled on a long gold rope, which opened worn velvet curtains that filled the wall from floor to ceiling. The heavy golden material parted dramatically, revealing nine large oil paintings. I glanced down at my one-page program. The paintings dated back to the 1920s, when Lawrence, known as a writer, had painted them in Europe. The paintings were confiscated in England for their erotic content. He was able to move them out of the country by promising they would stay in America. His benefactor was the owner of the La Fonda Hotel.

"I moved toward the paintings and their primitive shapes. I saw a range of naked buttocks, thighs, pubic hair; male-female parts. The paintings drew me in. The colors were somehow New Mexican desert colors, although he painted many of them in Italy.

"I realized that Lawrence had been a sexual rebel in his time, surrounded by negative publicity for *Lady Chatterley's Lover.* I smiled. The paintings were so benign compared to the pornography of today. If these paintings were done by a contemporary artist, they could hang safely and uncensored in any New York gallery today.

"When I got ready to leave, the guide standing by my side slowly closed the heavy drapes over this piece of 'erotic' art history. I asked her about the curtains.

"'Are they there to protect the pieces from dust and light? Or are they there to hide the content of the art?'

"She answered, 'Well, the governor was here last week, and the paintings are somewhat … .' She hesitated. I knew she was thinking, 'They are somewhat erotic.'

"Obviously, the paintings were not for public consumption. These erotic works would be hidden forever."

This story is an illustration of how erotic and beautiful the world is. All of our great artists and writers have understood the sensuality and eroticism of the world, and captured the interplay of lovers through their art.

My Client also realized that her own erotic life had been behind curtains of her own making for years, and now she was ready to open them up and share herself more honestly with her partner.

Censorship, sexism, views of women, economics, and politics have all played social roles in how we view eroticism and sexuality throughout our culture and how we create art depicting it. They have also shaped our beliefs about sex and kept us from being able to talk about it. Like golden curtains drawn over our fantasies, we hide our most private thoughts, even from those we love.

What would it be like to open the curtains and reveal the beauty of your own inner erotic life? Can you visualize yourself as someone who stands in the face of shame and explores his or her own sexual honesty?

The Differences between Male and Female Arousal

When we talk about arousal and our partners' bodies, we also include a discussion about the differences between men and women. There are similarities in sensitivity and orgasm, but there are also significant differences.

Because we don't always understand the differences between the sexes, there can be a lack of understanding in couples and a gap in sexual communication. It is easier to communicate what we need and want with our partners if our partners understand the differences between our bodies.

It takes women an average of eight to twenty minutes of direct clitoral stimulation to achieve orgasm, and yet when men were surveyed they thought it should take women no more than four minutes. This is not surprising in an age when women are faking orgasms at an average rate of seven out of every ten. If women fake an orgasm after four minutes, doesn't it reinforce for men that women only need four minutes of clitoral stimulation to orgasm?

EXERCISE
Mutual Sexual Awareness

The following exercise is a great way to begin to understand the differences between your body and your partner's. Your arousal cycle may be different from your partner's. It may take longer for your partner to get to a peak arousal phase where he or she is ready for orgasm. Understanding how your partner masturbates can teach you a tremendous amount about his or her sexual response cycle.

There is a lot of shame and embarrassment in our society around masturbation. Religious and cultural prohibitions about it have made the act of self-pleasure secret and hidden. Some people may feel more inhibited about masturbation than others. Women are sometimes more embarrassed about masturbating in front of a partner than men are, but differences in personality and personal sexual history have more to do with comfort levels than gender does. If you have grown up with prohibitions against masturbation, it might be hard to share this most personal of acts with another person.

Masturbating in front of our partners is like giving them instructions. It is a fast and wonderfully erotic way to increase the intimacy between the two of you. It gives you a physical language of sexual expression that tells more about your body than words can. Watching you touch yourself in ways that give you pleasure may be so arousing to your partner that it becomes an erotic encounter as well as a learning experience. It takes a lot of sexual generosity and understanding to give this gift of erotic connection to your partner.

First, before we can masturbate in front of our partner, we may need to find a mutual language that helps us break the ice. Getting over the discomfort and awkwardness around masturbation starts with a conversation. Communication about masturbation can be a turn-on, and it can be a way to connect to your partner. Now, with your Imago dialogue skills, you have a way to talk with your partner about what might otherwise be an uncomfortable topic.

For this exercise, you will need thirty minutes of safe, uninterrupted time. Because this may bring up some embarrassment, or even shame, privacy is essential. Find a place where you will not be interrupted and where there is a comfortable place to sit or lie down facing each other. Have this conversation in a safe and respectful way by giving each other the time and space to talk, and mirror back what the other has said. This is a great time to use validation and empathy in your dialogue. It will help your partner feel understood, and is the first step toward feeling safe.

Step One

Decide who will be the sender and who will be the receiver. Senders will talk for fifteen minutes about masturbation, and everything they can think of about the subject of self-pleasure. The receivers will mirror, always asking, "Is there more?"

For instance, ideas about masturbation might include how you feel about it, how often you do it, how you do it, what you were taught about it, and so on. Make sure you take the full fifteen minutes.

Step Two

Receivers mirror back what the senders have said, after each sentence or chunk. If they send too much, the receivers should ask them to send it over in smaller chunks so they can make sure they got it all.

Step Three

Receivers summarize, validate, and empathize. For example, the receiver might say, "So let me see if I got all that (summarize here to the best of your ability everything the sender has said about masturbation). It makes sense that you would feel this way about masturbation, knowing you the way I know you, because ... ."

(continued on page 108)

(continued)

Then check that out with the sender.

Receiver: "Did I get that?"

Sender: "You got me" or "Yes, and I want to make sure you heard the part where I said … ."

The receiver mirrors back if there was a part the sender wanted to make sure was heard.

Now empathize. It might sound like, "So it would make sense to me from everything you said that you would feel (include feeling words here like "removed, scared, anxious"). Are there other feelings you have that I didn't get?"

Sender: "No, you got me" or "Yes, I also feel … ."

The receiver then mirrors back any other feelings the sender has.

Step Four

Then you switch and the receiver becomes the sender.

Does it feel more likely that you would now feel comfortable enough with each other to masturbate in front of your partner? If so, make a date to do so.

Plan on a night where you will be undisturbed for an evening. Set the stage for an erotic evening. Take a long hot bath, wear sexy lingerie, light candles, and put soft sheets on the bed. Then pile up comfortable pillows, make sure you have lots of lubricant, and sit across from each other, where you can watch your partner while he or she watches you.

Moving from Sexual Curiosity to Erotic Action

6

Erotic curiosity is about thoughts, fantasies, and desires of a sexual or erotic nature. All mammals are sexual, but we are the only mammals that "eroticize" sex because we have the power to use our imagination to create erotic thoughts and images, which we use to fuel our passion.

Everyone has this capacity, although sometimes it may be difficult to get in touch with our fantasies. Some people engage in an active and erotic fantasy life, and some of us shut down our capacity for fantasy, and even get so rusty at it that we forget how. A healthy and active fantasy life is part of being a healthy and active human. Keeping the imagination alive helps keep our sex life alive and awake.

As we explore our erotic imagination and fantasy, this knowledge can help us communicate to our partner what we find exciting and stimulating. Using the Imago dialogue, we have skills that allow us to talk about our inner life and feel more intimate and connected to our partner.

There is a spectrum of normal human erotic curiosity. Understanding our personal spectrum of erotic thoughts can help us discover our fantasies and begin to make them happen.

Our erotic imagination includes three things—**curiosity, fantasy,** and **erotic action.** These three areas are all on an Erotic Curiosity Spectrum. The Erotic Curiosity Spectrum is a way to describe thoughts, fantasies, and desires on a continuum, from simple thoughts about sexual experiences to actions.

Erotic Curiosity Spectrum

Curiosity   Fantasy   Actions

At the left end of the spectrum are erotic thoughts about things we are curious about. These may include sex acts, erotic games, wearing sexy clothes, or wondering about what it would be like to have sex with other people, including friends, colleagues, or movie stars. Being erotically curious about something or someone doesn't necessarily mean we have full-blown fantasies about it; these are sometimes just passing thoughts or images. Maybe we have read about a sex act or have seen something in a movie that intrigues us, but we don't think much about it, or give it much energy. Still, there is a curiosity and a wondering.

Anything on your own erotic curiosity spectrum is normal for you. What you think about in the privacy of your mind is your own personal, fantastic movie theater on the screen of your imagination. What you do about your thoughts and fantasies are called erotic actions.

In the following exercises you will begin to explore your erotic curiosity, and then share your fantasies with your partner. Discovering these parts of yourself, you may find that your sexual desires become more intense. You will also be able to differentiate between what you would like to keep at a fantasy level and what you would like to take into action. Beginning to share these thoughts and feelings with your partner may feel scary or uncomfortable at first. Using the Imago dialogue, including mirroring, validating, and empathizing, can make it safer.

EXERCISE
From Sexual Curiosity to Erotic Action

There are several parts to this exercise, and you can do them all in one sitting, or you can do one part of the exercise and then leave it for a few days. There is no right or wrong way to do this. The important thing is that you explore some of your own inner fantasies and then share them with your partner using the Imago dialogue process.

You will start off with a writing exercise, which you do on your own. You are exploring your own erotic curiosity, and later you will dialogue with your partner about the things you have written.

Before you begin, find something to write on and a pen or pencil. You will need a comfortable place to sit and quiet time to think where you will not be interrupted.

These exercises will wake up your imagination and help you discover your deepest desires.

Step One

Write down three sexual things you are curious about, have wondered about, or want to know more about.

Step Two

The things that you wrote about in step one will naturally lead to thinking about your sexual fantasies.

The higher the level of curiosity, the more likely that there will be a fantasy about that erotic need. In other words, something you are curious about may eventually be something you fantasize about. Erotic curiosity can lead to fantasy.

Fantasies are thoughts and pictures in our minds that turn us on. They can be of people, sex acts, or erotic scenes. Things that make us feel sexy and erotic fall into this category.

For this part of the exercise, you will continue with a personal writing exercise, and this you do on your own. You are beginning to explore your personal erotic fantasies; later in this exercise you will have the opportunity to share this in a dialogue with your partner.

Before you begin, find something to write on and a pen or pencil. You will still need a comfortable place to sit and quiet time to think where you will not be interrupted.

Write down three things that you fantasize about.

1. Sometimes I fantasize about … .

2. There are times I get turned on when I think about … .

3. One thing I think is really hot is … .

Sometimes we share these things with our partners, letting them in on our fantasy life. And many times we keep our fantasies a secret. These fantasies may come to mind when we masturbate or when we have sex with our partners, but we don't necessarily talk about them.

(continued on page 112)

(continued)

Sometimes we find enough security in our relationship and we do talk to our partners about our fantasies, but we still don't act them out. They stay on a fantasy level only and serve as erotic energy or fuel for our sexuality.

Step Three

This next part of the exercise is about taking our fantasies into action. First write down fantasies you have that you might want to make come true. For example:

"My fantasy that I want to take into action is for me to hang on a swing from the ceiling and make love to my partner while suspended."

Then think about any props you might need, or special setting, or how you might need your partner to participate. Examples might be as follows:

Three things I need to make that happen are

1. I need to buy the swing.
2. I need my partner to help me screw it into the ceiling.
3. I need encouragement from him to make it happen.

Hold on to your answers and to your newfound clarity. Be excited and congratulate yourself that you have gotten this far! You are on the road to getting the sex you want.

Step Four

This next step is about sharing the fantasy that you want to take into action with your partner using the Imago dialogue. There is no need to commit to these things as you are listening to your partner express his or her desires.

This is different from an action plan; you don't have to agree or disagree at this time. Instead, the Imago dialogue offers a way to hold our partners in an active listening place, so they feel listened to and their desires are honored.

Expressing your desires and sharing the things you want to do with your partner can be a risk. You might be worried that your partner will not understand your desires, or will have different fantasies than you. You should hope so! Having a variety of desires and fantasies keeps a relationship exciting, and the thrill of discovering your partner's most secret fantasies can be incredibly erotic.

You may feel anxious about being so open, and this may make you feel vulnerable. Being vulnerable is good! It creates more intimacy. The more risk you take in trusting your partner with this valuable information, the more intense the connection will be between the two of you. Remember, hearing about your partner's fantasy can be a turn-on for you and telling his fantasy can be a turn-on for him. Do not under-estimate the power of sexual communication. It is an erotic life force that creates new energy and aliveness in your relationship.

Make sure you will have privacy for this exercise, and you may want to set up the room you are in for potential lovemaking after you are through. Turn on low lights or candles, and put on sexy clothes or lingerie. Take a bath or shower and shave before this exercise. Light incense or put fresh flowers close by. Using all of your senses will heighten the intensity of the sensual experience for both of you.

Find a comfortable place to sit for at least forty minutes or longer with your partner. Sit or lie down close enough to each other so that you can read notes that you made in the previous part of this exercise. If you are sitting across from each other, make sure you make eye contact. Sit with your knees touching as you face each other. The close proximity will increase the feeling of intimacy and connection.

Decide who will be the sender and who will be the receiver. The sender goes first.

Sender: "One thing I have fantasized about and would like to make happen is handcuffing you." (Describe your fantasy in as much detail as you can. What does it look like, feel like, smell like, taste like, sound like?)

Receiver (mirroring): "So one thing you have fantasized about that you would like to make happen is handcuffing me. Did I get that?"

Sender: "Yes" or "Let me make sure you got this part … ."

Receiver (mirroring): "Is there more?"

Sender: "No, you got it" or "Yes, and another thing is … ."

Sender: "Three things I would need to make this fantasy happen are a, b, and c."

Receiver (mirroring): "The three things you would need to make this fantasy happen are a, b, and c. Is there more?"

Sender: "No, you got it" or "Yes, another thing is … ."

Receiver (validating): "It makes sense to me that you would fantasize about … Knowing you the way I know you, it makes sense that you would want … ."

Receiver (empathizing): "And I can imagine that you would feel … if you were to have that fantasy come true."

Sender: "Yes, I would feel that" or "Yes, and I would also feel … ."

Now the sender and receiver switch.

(continued on page 114)

(continued)

When a fantasy is shared with your partner, it can raise the heat and passion between you, just by talking about it. Once a fantasy is out in the open between you, it can become something you talk about often, or just use on special occasions.

Step Five

Now comes the action plan. Find a quiet place for you and your partner to talk, facing one another. Decide who will be the sender and who will be the receiver.

Sender: "I would really like to make this fantasy happen within the next day/week/ month (choose a specific time frame)."

Receiver: "So you would really like to make this fantasy happen within the next day/week/month."

Sender: "Yes, if we did that it would make me feel … ."

Receiver (mirrors): "So if we did that it would make you feel … (validates): It makes sense to me that you would want to do this within a day/month/year. (empathizes): I imagine that if we did that you would feel … ."

Sender: "You got me" or "I also want you to know I would feel … ."

As you close this exercise, add an appreciation at the end and then switch. This is a wonderful way to end an exercise that might be a high risk for both of you. Appreciation is a very validating and emotionally responsive reaction to any high-risk sharing. It gives a nice closure and adds an important element that can become an ongoing part of your conversations.

Now that you have shared the fantasy that you would like to take into action, begin to create that reality. Don't wait for your partner to provide the catalyst for your fantasy. Begin to explore what you need to make the fantasy happen.

Over the next few weeks, begin to think about your fantasy as something that you are coming closer to. Let the erotic tension build as you look forward to making it happen.

The Consequences of Making Fantasies Come True

Acting out a fantasy or curiosity can be great, or it can be painful for you or others. Actions can be healthy or not, depending on your relationship and how they affect your partner. Our actions always have consequences.

If we have a fantasy about having an affair and act it out, for example, this action usually affects all those involved. (See more about affairs below.)

What we choose to take from fantasy to action should be determined by our personal boundaries and a sense of integrity. An example of this might be a fantasy that is common to both men and women—the ménage à trois, or threesome. Both men and women fantasize about adding a third person to their lovemaking at some point in their relationship. Taking this fantasy into action may have many consequences. And sometimes the reality is not as good as the fantasy!

Threesomes can be exciting and sexy, but the reality is that they can also be messy, awkward, and emotionally threatening. Talking about this fantasy without acting it out can spice up your sex life, with no negative consequences to the relationship.

Being clear with your lover that you have a fantasy you would like to share but are not ready to take to the action stage can actually make it easier to share the fantasy. When you tell your partner about your fantasy, you can always preface the conversation with a request. Indicate whether you would like to keep the fantasy as a fantasy or whether you want to act it out. Knowing that your partner will more clearly understand where your fantasy falls on the Erotic Curiosity Spectrum can prevent feeling pressure to act it out before you are ready. For example, you might be more likely to share your fantasy of being suspended from the ceiling during sex if you are not worried that your partner will run out right away and buy hooks to hang you from!

(continued on page 116)

The Consequences of Making Fantasies Come True (continued)

Sharing your fantasies with a lover falls on the right, or more active, side of the spectrum. When you choose not to share some of your erotic curiosity with your partner, then these thoughts fall on the left, or passive, side of the spectrum.

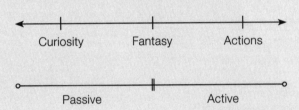

Erotic Curiosity Spectrum

Curiosity   Fantasy   Actions

Passive   Active

Submissive versus Dominant

Also on the erotic curiosity spectrum are two general categories—receptive and directive. Our thoughts and fantasies run toward a preference to be receptive or controlled in bed. Being under someone's erotic control falls on the submissive side of the spectrum.

Or we might have thoughts and fantasies about being more dominant or directive and like the idea of being able to be in erotic control of our partner. Both of these categories function as their own erotic spectrum, with many variations of control, and the erotic power plays of submission and domination can be acted out in many ways.

Erotic Curiosity Spectrum

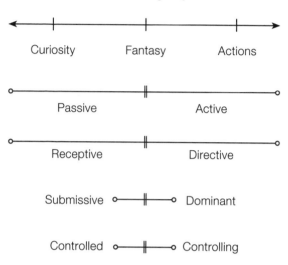

Consider what's on your erotic curiosity spectrum. Are you more turned on by thoughts of being receptive, sexually controlled, and submissive? Sexual submissives might enjoy thoughts of being told what to do or being spanked.

If you are sexually directive and enjoy thoughts of being in control sexually, you may have more dominant fantasies, including being on top during missionary sex, blindfolding your partner, or "ordering" your partner to perform oral sex.

This part of the exercise will help you decide which fantasy you want to make happen in your relationship. Any thoughts that have moved from curiosity to fantasy, which you now would like to begin to explore, can be included in this "action" area. These fantasies can be reasonable, where all the practical aspects of acting out the fantasy seem simple and obtainable, or they can be complicated and take planning and communication to make them happen.

In both cases, taking a fantasy into action can be thrilling and exciting—or somewhat disappointing. Sometimes things are best left as fantasy. And for others, acting out your most private thoughts and desires can be the pinnacle of joy and connection in your relationship.

A Catalyst to Move Fantasies into Action

Moving fantasies from the imagination end of the spectrum to the action end of the spectrum can be a big leap for some couples. It might be very comfortable to have a fantasy that stays in the imagination. Perhaps you share this with your partner. Being clear with him or her that you are just sharing a fantasy is different than asking your partner to help live out that fantasy in real life.

Sometimes we need a catalyst to have our fantasies come to fruition. That catalyst might be anything that pushes us from curiosity to fantasy to *action*.

Many times we need a stimulus to help us act out our fantasies. A catalyst might mean being in the right place at the right time. Or it might mean our partner makes something happen for us that convinces us to move forward into action.

An example of this type of stimulus is reflected in the following couple's case.

Anne came into my office complaining that her sex life was dull and unimaginative. She shared that she always had orgasms, but that she felt bored with sex and wanted to try something new with her husband, Tim.

Using the erotic curiosity exercises, she wrote down the things that she was curious about, the things she fantasized about, and the fantasies that she wanted to take into action.

Through this exercise she discovered that she was curious about dressing up in costumes and role-playing during sex. She always wondered how people made those things happen, and she was wondering whether she would have the energy and courage to present this curiosity to her partner.

She wrote down her thoughts and realized that she often fantasized about dressing up in a maid's outfit. She thought about this for several days and nights, and fantasized about what it would be like to be waiting for her partner when he came home from work at night, wearing a black and white maid's costume and holding a dustpan. She found herself turned on by these fantasies. Anne then decided she wanted to take this fantasy into action. But, she wasn't sure she could make it happen on her own.

She shared her fantasy with her partner, Tim, and using the dialogue process he was able to mirror, validate, and empathize. Still, Anne couldn't move her fantasy into action. She was delighted that Tim could talk about it with her, and for a while that added a new energy and enthusiasm to their lovemaking.

One day she came home from her job and found on her bed a maid's outfit, complete with feather duster and dustpan. The skirt was short, and there was a ruffled apron and a tight top with a name tag that said "Anne" pinned to the front.

This was the catalyst she needed. She was able to put on the costume and play the part of the maid, and she waited for her husband to come into the bedroom that evening, where she was dressed in costume and able to act out her fantasy.

EXERCISE
Be Your Own Catalyst

After you have discussed your fantasy, find one thing that represents your fantasy—let this be something of your own choosing.

Perhaps it is a piece of clothing, an accessory, or a sex toy. Buy this item, bring it into your home, and keep it in your bedroom to remind you of your fantasy.

Giving the Go-Ahead
Sometimes we need permission to act out our fantasies.

It is hard for women in particular to ask for what they want sexually. Because of the guilt and shame attached to sexual desire for women, it can be hard to own the need for sex. Some women say they don't have the self-esteem or the confidence to ask for their erotic fantasies to be fulfilled. Even if they are curious about

(continued on page 120)

(continued)

something, they might not feel they have the right to ask for it. It is important for women to own their desires, to state them clearly, and to let go of the guilt and shame about asking for what they want.

It can also be scary for men to ask for their desires and fantasies to be fulfilled. Men are sometimes more articulate about asking for action than they are about expressing emotion. Women can sometimes speak more freely about their feelings, but find it difficult to talk about what they want in bed.

Asking our partner to help us take our fantasies from imagination to action can be hard for both sexes. Getting permission first, or waiting for a catalyst to make something happen, can ensure that we have an easier time with it. But the most direct way to begin to live our fantasy sex life is to share with our partner what our fantasies are and which ones we want to make happen.

EXERCISE
Commitment to Focus

Committing to working on one fantasy can bring focus to our relationships. It gives erotic energy a chance to grow and develop. The fantasy becomes the catalyst for change in the relationship. And committing to creating this new fantasy together gives the partnership a common goal and a focus on growth.

For the following exercise, you need a piece of paper and a pen. Think about one sexual aspect of your partnership that you want to focus on for a finite period of time. Decide how long you want to completely focus on that one aspect. For example, this could mean having intercourse every night for a certain, limited amount of time. It may mean that you try all the exercises in this book over a long weekend.

Share your idea with your partner and listen to your partner's idea. Is there a common goal that you can both work toward?

Decide what your commitment will be to each other and sign the sexual contract below:

I, [insert name], am totally committed to our sexual relationship for the next [insert specific time frame]. This includes being totally faithful, and focusing all my energy on pleasing you. I am committed to exploring your erotic fantasies for this amount of time. I will also [fill in blank].

Leave the contract somewhere you can both see it. Check in periodically (e.g., daily or weekly) to see how you are doing. Are there consequences in your partnership for not living up to your commitments? What are they?

Why Fantasies Happen

Fantasies happen for a reason. Fantasies are a direct result of our anxieties and fears. We work out our anxieties through our sexuality.

What we fantasize about is also many times our psychological edge. An "edge" is the place at the end of our comfort zone. It is a line where we feel comfortable on one side, and uncomfortable on the other. But we will be stuck if we stay where we are. Picture a plant growing against a windowpane, searching for fresh air and sunshine. The "edge" for the plant is the window. It would like to move beyond its comfort zone, but may not know how to get there. Pushing against our edge in our sexuality means moving into the places where we initially feel uncomfortable, but ultimately more whole and fulfilled.

In our sexuality, we all have psychological needs. For example, we have a need to feel safe, a need to feel loved, and a need to feel excited and turned on. We also have psychological fears, such as the feeling of being trapped, the fear of heights, or the fear of abandonment.

We fantasize about things that are on our psychological edge. Many times our sexual fantasies are also our psychological and relational fears. This psychological anxiety can make sex tantalizing. If we are excited about something that causes us stress, we experience it as a thrill. Think of a roller coaster or skydiving. They may feel dangerous and scary, but we are also highly stimulated and excited when we do those things. Sometimes our fantasies give us that "rush" as well.

When Forbidden Acts Become Fantasies

We seek mastery over our fears though our sexual fantasies. This is an interesting way that our minds work to heal us of our greatest anxieties. Through seeking pleasure and stimulation, we can turn something scary and negative into something arousing and beautiful. The forbidden becomes fantasy, and we have the power through our imaginations to have a sense of control over our deepest worries. We can control, in our minds, who does what to whom, how long it lasts, and how it ends. This gives us sense of mastery over the things we feel we have no control over.

These forbidden aspects of desire make our fantasies rich and alive.

Forbidden acts can become fantasies, and with enough safety and communication between partners, they can become part of our sex life.

An example of how our anxiety becomes fantasy is illustrated in the case below. Notice how acting out the fantasy actually heals Tara of her persistent and chronic fears.

Using Sex to Overcome Anxiety

Tara came into my office complaining of anxiety. She suffered from claustrophobia, a fear of small spaces. When asked if she had any other fears, she admitted she also had entrapment fears in her relationships. If she felt emotionally "trapped" in a commitment to a partner, she would react by feeling some panic, clenching her teeth, and sweating. This was the same response she experienced in elevators. After many years, she was finally in a relationship with a man she was able to commit to and not panic when she felt trapped.

Tara's concern was that she was having sexual fantasies that were disturbing to her. The erotic fantasies she had were about being trapped! She felt herself being turned on by thoughts of not having control during sex, such as being tied up, handcuffed, or held down. She fantasized about her boyfriend playing a dominant role during sex and ordering her to lie down and take her clothes off. She had fantasies about being restricted. It felt counter intuitive for her to feel erotically charged over being trapped, while at the same time having entrapment fears. She wanted desperately to tell her partner that she had these thoughts, but didn't know how. Her shame was too overwhelming.

She was confused about why she felt turned on by something she found so disturbing in the rest of her life. It was understandable that Tara would feel confused about her fantasies. What was distressing to her was also a turn-on. Her confusion was about whether she should seek pleasure in this way, given that this same area brought her such distress. What she needed to experience was how her fantasy of being trapped could actually decrease her fears and anxiety.

Her intuition (and her therapy) told her that if she could begin to talk about her fears, they would lessen. She trusted her partner, Bill, and wanted to talk with him about her fantasies. She also understood that to feel totally fulfilled, she would like to take this fantasy into action with Bill. After doing the exercises on erotic curiosity, she began to explore what she had written. She wrote about the things she was erotically curious about, what she fantasized about, and what she wanted to take into action. She knew she would need Bill's support and understanding and found she was anticipating a dialogue with Bill about her fantasy. She waited for the right moment with great trepidation and also a heightened sense of erotic stimulation.

Soon Tara found the time to share her fantasy with her partner. Bill had done the exercise on erotic curiosity as well, and he was excited to share his fantasies with Tara. Tara went first, and was the sender. Bill listened to what she had to say. He did not try to comfort her as she talked, but just mirrored everything she had to tell him.

Tara: "So, I know its crazy, but I have this fantasy that you will tie me to the bed. And that I won't be able to get out. And you will have sex with me while I am trapped there. I know that's awfully strange, since I have such a fear of being trapped!"

Bill: "So, let me see if I got this. You have a fantasy that I will tie you to the bed." Bill gazed into Tara's eyes as he mirrored back to her and she visibly relaxed in her chair. "And you think about what it would be like to not be able to get out. You want me to have sex with you while you are trapped there on the bed. You think it's awfully strange to have this fantasy since you have such a fear of being trapped. Did I get it all?"

Tara: "Yes, perfectly."

Eventually, Bill and Tara did act out this fantasy. Bill tied her to his bed with silk scarves. She felt excited and could feel her heart race and her pulse increase. She also experienced some anxiety mixed in with sexual excitement. Bill and Tara had sex while she was tied up. She experienced a deep and profound orgasm.

The next day, as she got on to an elevator, she felt some anxiety, but also to her amazement, she felt pleasure. What she hadn't expected was that acting out her sexual fantasy would change the experiences in the rest of her life.

Her body remembered that being "trapped" wasn't all that bad. She had worked through some of her entrapment fears by acting them out in bed.

This makes sense. Tara did something she was afraid of, which was now connected to deep pleasure. She was able to control her entrapment by asking Bill to do it, by giving him permission to tie her up, and by letting him have sex with her while she was bound. She could have stopped the game at any time, and she knew that Bill would honor that. She had created a scenario that gave her power over her fears. Her anxiety was now something she had control of.

The act of working out this fantasy in life actually connected a pleasure stimulus to the anxiety, in a safe and erotically charged moment, with a loving partner. This created a positive connection in her mind with a positive physical experience, and the feeling of being trapped in other areas of her life could now be experienced differently.

The Fear Factor

Fear is a powerful motivator. It keeps us stuck and locked into patterns of relating to others that is not always in our best interest. We may freeze and cut off parts of ourselves that need expression, or we may act out in ways that are defenses against being overwhelmed by our fear.

There are healthier ways to deal with our fears. We can use the Imago method to communicate and express our fear. Imago gives us the language to share our anxieties and hope for a better way.

The following case example describes a couple exploring fear in this new way. Although it feels risky to share with a partner something we are afraid of, this can actually increase our intimacy and connection with our partner. Sharing our fears lessens their intensity, and it also helps us look at fear in a new way.

Jenna and Mark had been in couple's therapy for a few sessions when they started talking about their sexual fantasies. They also talked honestly about their fears. Jenna's worst fear, because of her childhood, was the psychological fear of abandonment. This manifested itself in her persistent fear that her husband was going to leave her for another woman. This was not based on anything he had actually done. Mark constantly reminded her that he was faithful and loved her deeply.

Jenna's fear of abandonment was also her most secret sexual fantasy. She found herself fantasizing about her husband having sex with another woman. She wanted to watch him while he went down on another woman, giving her an orgasm through oral sex. She thought about this often but was too afraid to tell her husband, for fear that he would act it out and fall in love with the other woman, and then leave her, as she had always feared.

Jenna was balanced on the precipice of fear and erotic energy. Her fantasy was for her husband to have sex with another woman. It was not to participate sexually with the two of them, but to watch the woman having oral sex with her husband. This felt like a psychological edge because it contained "danger" for her.

As mentioned previously, an "edge" is the place where we most resist change. We all have boundaries, socially and sexually. Our edge is also the place where we need to grow the most. When we push our edge, even just slightly, we grow into areas that are new for us, which allows us to experience more joy and fulfillment.

Sometimes pushing our edge can be a real stretch. The way we grow sexually by slowly pushing the boundaries of what we are comfortable with. These stretches also help us to push our edges and grow into the people we need to be.

Stretching into places that hold anxiety for us is many times exactly what our partner is asking us to do. Sometimes those places are the hardest for us to grow into. Stretching for our partner could mean sharing our deepest thoughts and feelings. It might mean sharing fantasies we have kept secret. It could even mean trying something new in bed because it's important to our partner. If our lover asks us to do something that feels like too big of a stretch, we can ask for a smaller stretch.

Jenna was pushing her edge by telling Mark about her fantasy. This was a scary and uncomfortable place, but she felt that in doing so she would grow closer to him and be a more confident sexual being.

Jenna and Mark were able to talk about the fantasy she had of watching him with another woman. They used the dialogue process to talk about it. Mark listened to Jenna describe her fantasy of seeing him in bed with someone else, and he mirrored back everything she said. After every revelation, he asked her, "Is there more?"

Because of his encouragement, Jenna was also able to share her confusion. She asked Mark to understand that although she thought about it, she was not convinced she wanted to bring her fantasy into the action phase.

When Mark listened to Jenna's fantasy and her fears, he validated her by saying things like this:

Mark: "Jenna, knowing you like I know you, it makes total sense to me that you would be nervous about taking that step to live out your fantasy. I can understand that this must be so difficult for you to talk about, since you have expressed your fears about me leaving you for someone else."

When Mark went on and empathized with her feelings, Jenna seemed to relax in her seat.

Mark: "I can imagine that talking about this makes you very nervous. It must be scary to confess these thoughts and fears. I also imagine that if you were to act out this fantasy you might feel very conflicted. It might turn you on, but also make you feel slightly insecure. Is there more?"

Jenna: "You got me. That's exactly how I would feel. And yes, it makes me nervous and uncomfortable to talk about these things. It also, to be honest, turns me on a little."

Mark: "Oh, okay, so it makes you nervous and uncomfortable to talk about these things, but it also turns you on a little? Did I get that?"

Jenna: "You got me." She giggled.

Mark: "Is there more?"

Jenna: "Well, I hope that we can agree to keep this fantasy just a fantasy for now."

Mark: "So you want to keep this fantasy just a fantasy for now."

He agreed, but he asked if they could talk about the fantasy again.

Sometimes fantasies can stay fantasies and not move to the action phase. Instead, the fantasy can be integrated into their lovemaking. For example, during sex Mark could whisper in Jenna's ear as they are having intercourse,

"If there was another woman here, I would go down on her and you could watch ... ." This would let Jenna play with the fantasy over time without feeling threatened.

As a result of sharing and playing with this fantasy together, Jenna realized that she no longer had the fear that Mark would leave her. She felt more connected to him and felt safer in their relationship than ever before. Mark was turned on just by hearing her fantasy. He was also so flattered that Jenna trusted him enough to share her fantasy with him that he felt more intimately connected to her.

If Jenna decided to take the fantasy to the action phase, she could live out her greatest fear and experience erotic pleasure. Over time she might deal with her fears about Mark differently. What she was most afraid of also gave her an erotic charge. Mark felt that someday they could safely act out her fantasy and still stay connected.

This couple confronted a fear that was also a fantasy, and the energy that was released from this sharing created a whole new dynamic in the relationship. They were able to work through jealousy and possessiveness and see them less as a threat to the relationship and more as a way to express tension and fear, and then work it out through sharing their deepest desires with one another. This case is also an example of how using the dialogue works for most, if not all, of our sexual issues in our partnerships.

Discovering Where Your Fantasies Fall on the Erotic Curiosity Spectrum

Below is a list of common fantasies that fall on both ends of the erotic curiosity spectrum. Sit with your partner and fill out this exercise separately, but in the same room.

Go down the list, and mark each item with a number from 1 through 5. When you are through, share your responses with your partner.

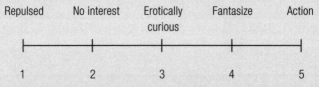

Repulsed	No interest	Erotically curious	Fantasize	Action
1	2	3	4	5

1. One means you are repulsed by the idea.
2. Two means the idea holds no interest for you.
3. Three means you are erotically curious about it.
4. Four means you have fantasies about it.
5. Five means you would like to turn this fantasy into action.

Examples of fantasies:

- Watching two women have sex
- Having sex with a man and a woman
- Having sex with your partner and another couple
- Multiple partner sex
- Having sex with a group of strangers
- Being seduced by an older woman
- Watching a woman masturbate
- Masturbating in front of your partner
- Being dominant with a woman
- Being dominated by a woman
- Receiving oral sex

- Receiving oral sex from your partner
- French kissing partner after a blow job
- Partner swallowing after a blow job
- Sex with a call girl or stripper
- Sex with a celebrity
- Sex with someone you know (not your partner)
- Receiving anal stimulation
- Having anal sex
- Tying up a woman and having sex with her
- Forcing your partner to have sex
- Forcing another woman to have sex
- Being forced to have sex
- Being filmed during sex
- Talking dirty
- Double penetration
- Watching pornography with your partner
- Acting out pornography scenes with your partner
- Anonymous sex with a stranger
- Sex with an old boyfriend/girlfriend
- Sex with another woman
- Sex with two men
- Sex with a group including your partner
- Sex with a group of men
- Sex in front of your partner with someone else
- Being dominated by your partner
- Being spanked
- Having toes sucked
- Sex with vegetables or fruit

(continued on page 130)

Discovering Where Your Fantasies Fall
on the Erotic Curiosity Spectrum (continued)

- Sex with food (e.g., whipped cream)
- Sex with vibrators and dildos
- Masturbating with vibrator in front of your partner
- Sex outside or in public places

Domination Fantasies:

- Dressing up in leather
- Role-playing with costumes (e.g., stripper, cowboy, doctor)
- Wearing boots or high heels
- Tying up your partner
- Putting handcuffs on your partner
- Putting a collar on your partner
- Pinching your partner with clothespins
- Using a cane, riding crop, or whip to threaten
- Using a cane, riding crop, or whip to inflict sensation
- Blindfolding your partner
- Having your partner lick your boots
- Urinating on your partner
- Sex doggie style
- Playing the master role
- Slave weekend*

Submission Fantasies:

- Dressing up in plastic
- Dressing up in rubber
- Dressing in women's clothes (for the man)

*Slave weekend is when you and your partner stay in the roles of master
and slave for two days, without breaking roles.

- Being urinated on
- Playing the slave role
- Being handcuffed
- Being tied up
- Being strapped down
- Wearing a collar
- Having your hair pulled
- Submitting and thanking partner
- Being caned or whipped
- Being spanked

Talk with your partner about what came up for you, what it feels like to hear his or her answers, and how you feel now that you have read and talked about your fantasies.

How Exits Take Us Away from Our Relationships

We all have behaviors that take our focus away from our love relationship, and sometimes we use these behaviors as a way to avoid intimacy or connection. "Exits" are ways in which we avoid being "present" or actively involved in our relationship. If we choose these "exits" we have to be aware of the consequences.

Some examples of exits include the following:

- Drinking excessively
- Using drugs
- Eating compulsively
- Shopping compulsively
- Over focusing on the children
- Spending excessive time at hobbies
- Using the computer or watching television to excess
- Watching pornography
- Having affairs
- Getting involved in Internet relationships
- Spending time in chat rooms
- Working too much
- Going out with friends
- Traveling
- Reading

Many of these exits could be behaviors that feel healthy and are not necessarily negative. Things like hobbies and focusing on our children are important and necessary, and they also help us grow as individuals. Some of these exits are behaviors that are fine in moderation, but when they are used to avoid intimacy, they can become problematic.

Affairs: Exits and the Invisible Divorce

Searching for a partner outside of our primary relationship can take us away from building on the relationship we have. Sometimes an affair can be an "exit" or an "invisible divorce." Often it can be a way to avoid the issues in our current partnership.

Feeling passion in your relationship means being thrilled that you want what you have. Energy going out of the relationship to other potential partners can drain the energy we have to focus on each other. Safety sometimes includes an understanding that no other sexual partners will be involved. For most couples, this safety in the relationship allows for open exploration of erotic fantasies.

An affair can take away our feeling of trust. However, an affair does not necessarily mean the relationship has to end. Most people have affairs not because there is something lacking in their relationship, but because an opportunity presents itself.

Making a choice to close your "exits" can increase the power flow into your current partnership. Instead of draining the focus off of our issues, the extra energy can help us figure out what we want. If there are people, places, or things that are draining your energy, can you identify them?

Read the list on page 131 and see if you can find what your exits are. Are there any exits you use that you can add to this list? Think about which of these you might be willing to modify or give up, at least temporarily.

More specifically, can you identify what exits you use to avoid focusing on your sexual partnership? Perhaps watching TV at night, reading in bed, staying at work late, drinking at night, or going out with your friends all interfere with the intimacy in your life.

Can you make a commitment to your current partner that for a finite period of time you will focus all of your energy on your emotional and sexual relationship? For a limited amount of time can you commit to closing at least one of your exits?

Is there one thing that you might be willing to give up for a month? For six weeks? Share these things with your partner and make a commitment to close one of these exits for a finite period of time. This will give you more energy to increase the passion in your partnership. It may also bring up other issues that you might be avoiding in your life. Maybe now is the time to look at them.

EXERCISE
Exit Contract

Use this contract to help you close one or more of these exits:

I, [name], am totally committed to closing the exit I use to avoid intimacy. The exit I will close is [name a specific exit]. I commit to closing this exit for the next [include specific time frame].

Signed _____

Now that you have taken this giant step toward change, what exactly do you want to focus on? What issues do you have that need to be looked at? What can you commit to doing for a finite period of time that will help work on this issue in your partnership? Perhaps you and your partner just want to work on improving your partnership on an erotic level. What is one thing that you think will help you do that?

Closing exits is about not doing something. Commitments are about doing something differently. Commitment means only that you make a decision. Think about what decisions you can make regarding your exits and where you can push your edge. Think about what your partner would appreciate now that you know more about his or her fantasies. What fantasies would you like to commit to working on?

Closing exits and committing to focus totally on the erotic aspect of your partnership creates a new safety in your relationship. The irony is that safety must exist to create an environment where vulnerability, fantasy, and risk can happen. This allows for greater passion and erotic sex. However, safety is sometimes antithetical to erotic sex. If erotic sex is illicit or forbidden, even in your imagination, then safety is not necessarily a turn-on! And yet safety needs to happen for partners to go to a deeper level sexually. Greater passion means greater depth and greater connection.

How to Safely Explore "Dark" Fantasies

Sometimes safety is being able to live out your deepest and perhaps darkest fantasies. Sometimes fantasies fall on the dominant side of the erotic curiosity spectrum, and sometimes they are on the submissive side. They may contain thoughts about bondage, domination, or submission.

For instance, many people have a picture in their minds of "S&M" or " sadism" and "masochism" as anonymous and involving black leather, full-face masks, pain, and torture. Another common picture of S&M is the dominatrix in black leather boots with a whip torturing the defenseless submissive tied to the floor.

These notions may all be true, but bondage, discipline, and sadomasochism, or BDSM, is more often about a range of play that includes varying levels of sensation. There is a wide range of true BDSM interests and participant levels. Partners play roles in the dominant/submissive (dom/sub) world of sexual play. Acting out scenes is a form of role-play where each partner feels safe enough to step into a part and act it out for each other.

In BDSM play, one partner is in the dominant role of "bossing" the other around for the pleasure of being in control. The submissive is giving "permission" to be used in that role. The dominant is acting out the role as a gift to the submissive partner. The other partner is submissive, taking pain or "punishment." This role-play can be foreplay or include penetration and orgasm.

The polarities of good and bad roles play with energy and power, transferring it from one person to the other and back again. These two ends of the spectrum can create a strong attraction or repulsion.

Acting Out Light Fantasies

Light fantasies are romantic and sweet scenarios that make you feel sexy. These fantasies may be more traditional than dark fantasies, but they are not necessarily better or worse. Some examples of light fantasies might include the following:

- Sensual massage with aromatherapy lotion
- Taking a warm bath together
- Making love on a bed of rose petals
- Making love by candlelight
- Listening to soothing music while making love
- Tickling each other with feather dusters
- Wearing lacy lingerie
- Using ice cubes
- Shaving one another
- Slow dancing in the dark

All of these fantasies can be combined with sex or experienced alone. Being mindful and in the moment adds passion to light moments. Breathing in to the moment and focusing completely on your partner can bring a heightened arousal of all your senses. Focus on what you smell: the candles, the bathwater, the rose petals, your partner's skin. Focus on what you hear: soft music, your partner's breathing, etc. Focus on what each of your senses is telling you, and give yourself permission to be totally relaxed in the moment.

Creating a Safe Word

Before a BDSM role-play, both partners should always commit to a "safe word." A "safe word" is a word decided on beforehand that is not something that one might normally say in the course of the play. This is a way to say "no" or "stop." Creating this word helps both partners feel more comfortable playing their roles.

One is likely to moan or scream things like "oh, God," "no, don't," or even "stop." But these words may be part of what keeps submissives in their role, and only part of the act. A real "safe word" would be something totally out of the ordinary for that moment, like "cherry pie" or "frog." It doesn't matter what the word is, as long as you both agree to it before the games begin.

Dominants need to know that they can continue the game, trusting submissives to end the play when they need to. The sexual tension that is created during the games should be part of the energy that grows between you. Remember that starting out at a high sensation level is not pleasant, and that most of us need to build up slowly to tolerate pain as well as pleasure. Working up to more intense sensation is the goal.

You might include toys in your BDSM play, such as handcuffs, blindfolds, leather cuffs, and collars. Sex toys include dildos, vibrators, anal plugs, and nipple clamps. Games include spanking, whipping, caning, and pinching the body with clothespins.

EXERCISE
Sexual Sending and Receiving

In this exercise, you will need at least sixty minutes of uninterrupted time and privacy. Create a sexy environment by darkening the room, lighting candles, and putting fresh flowers by the bed. Put clean, soft sheets and blankets on the bed or floor where you will be. Put on soft, sexy music in the background. Take the time to create an erotic environment you will both enjoy. This is a way to honor your sexual relationship and bring a level of integrity and respect to your lovemaking.

Find props before you begin. You will need several long silk scarves. Take the phone off the hook and begin.

Step One

First, decide who will be receptive (receiver) and who will be directive (sender). Senders should start by kissing their lover softly and slowly, and then become more assertive in their kisses. Lift your partner's arms above her head and continue kissing her on her neck and chest.

Step Two

Gently and seductively, tie her hands above her head with a silk scarf, being careful not to cut off circulation. Tie another silk scarf over her eyes. Continue to kiss, lick, and nibble her body with her hands tied and eyes blindfolded. Make love to your partner without asking how she wants it. Love her in ways that you know will please both of you.

Step Three

Afterward, take off the silk scarves slowly and hold your partner quietly for several moments. Give her a chance to come down from the experience and reconnect with you. Discuss what the experience was like for both of you.

Step Four

Next time, reverse roles.

Playing the Game

Spanking is a very intimate form of "light" BDSM. It is more intimate than other types of BDSM because there is lots of bodily contact. It also triggers the release of endorphins, the feel-good brain chemicals released under stress.

Spanking, done with an open hand or palm, can be a way to inflict a sensation that becomes pleasurable for the submissive partner, and it gives the dominant partner a feeling of control. There is also a temporary visual mark left on the buttocks. The pinkness is sometimes called "pinking" the submissive. Always remember that gentler is better! Start slowly and lightly.

To begin, the submissive person can be lying down, kneeling, or tied up with rope, handcuffs, or scarves. The dominant person should decide how the submissive will be restricted, being very careful not to cut off circulation. Remember that as the submissive pulls on the ropes or cuffs, they may get tighter, so allow for some room to prevent blood flow restriction.

(continued on page 138)

Playing the Game (continued)

Make the restriction part of the game. Dominant partners, or "tops" should take their time, making sure that the submissive partners, or "bottoms," feel every moment of the tension that is building as they get more and more helpless. The rope or cuffs can be slid over the submissive's body parts, so he experiences the delightful titillation of knowing what is to come when he is restricted.

A blindfold works well to heighten the sexual tension and leave the submissive guessing about what's coming next. Differing levels of sensation can be created now. Slowly, the top can begin teasing by touching, pinching, or squeezing all parts of the bottom's body. Levels of pain can be increased as the bottom becomes more used to the sensation. The slight pain of gentle pinches or taps can be increased as the bottom gets more turned on.

Using a small whip or cane, the top can inflict gentle whipping or caning, starting softly. Remember, this is all about sensation. A harder stroke or a stronger squeeze will be perceived in the same way. As the endorphins increase and the bottom becomes more accustomed to the teasing pain, then harder strokes can be used.

Some strokes will leave a mark or redness on the body, and this can be a turn-on for the top. Alternate between harder and harder sensations and softer, soothing strokes.

The top can whisper in the partner's ear all the things she wants to do to him. This can make the bottom swoon with anticipation.

The top can be in control and have power over the partner in this way. The bottom in this game can relax and let go, knowing the top is in charge. This allows the bottom to totally relax and enjoy, and it gives both roles the erotic connection they may be looking for. The direct connection between demanding what you want and getting what you want is a powerful feeling. Erotic requests made with clear instructions and permission increases the feeling of control and safety for the bottom.

This permission often allows both partners to feel empowered. Without having to manipulate to get what they want, they can act it out. And this game can be acted out over and over again! The capacity to be fully present for the game and to escape reality by going totally into sensation is the lure of BDSM.

Use caution with this exercise. It takes very little pressure to create a sensation. The back of a brush, a riding crop, or a bamboo rod can all create the sensation of a hard spanking or "caning."

Always remember to choose a safe word before you start. Remember, whichever role you're in, you both carry great responsibility in creating safety while tolerating greater levels of intensity.

For this exercise, you will need at least sixty minutes, and lots of privacy. Make sure you will not be interrupted, either by children, the phone or other distractions. Safety and security are particularly important in this exercise.

Be highly tuned in to the needs of the submissive. Show empathy by mirroring their sounds or mirroring their words in your mind. Listen carefully to their breathing and their sounds of pleasure or fear. Be particularly sensitive to feelings that come up before, during, and after this exercise. This may push partners to the edge of their comfort zone, and extra affection may be in order after you are through. Be prepared to be affectionate and loving when you are through, and do this in any way that makes you feel appreciative of your partner. Stroke her physically, being soft and comforting with your hands. Talk softly in her ear and reassure her that you love and care for her, and that she is safe. This experience can be very powerful, because it is a high intensity exercise and can bring up confusion for many couples.

The most important part of this exercise is to have fun with it! Remember that playing erotic games is part of finding joy and intensity in your sex life. This is a role-play game as well as a game of sensation and intensity. Experience the pleasure of being the "top" and also the power of being the "bottom."

Talk after this exercise if you need to, or drift into sleep, knowing that talking later may feel important and necessary.

Caning

To do this exercise, the bottoms, or subs, should be bent over a table, ottoman, or the other person's lap—somewhere that they can be comfortable for a while.

Starting slowly, tap the buttocks with a rhythmic percussion. Increase your speed before you increase the intensity. Eventually, the buttocks will adjust to the sensation and some numbness might result. Harder caning will produce a greater release of endorphins and the bottom may experience more painful strokes as pure sensation. You can alternate your strokes with harder slaps of the cane and break the pattern, creating tension as the bottom or sub waits for the next tap.

Always stop when the bottom, or sub, says his or her safe word.

When you are ready, help the bottom come out of the experience gently.

Remember to go slowly to help the bottom transition from the intensity of the experience. Show affection and support in a low and calming voice.

If this exercise leads to sex, enjoy it! Have fun with the endorphins that have been released, and remember that all sensations can be pleasurable.

The Submissive

Submissives temporarily give up control of their worlds during sex. There is a freedom in having someone else take erotic control of the body.

For some, being submissive during sex or BDSM play can be a healing experience. Allowing someone else to take the control gives subs permission to totally let go, to surrender. Letting someone dominate completely allows that surrender, stretching beyond the openings of the body and into the psychological strongholds of the mind.

For women, the need to surrender during sex is connected to the physiological need to "let go" in order to orgasm. Women often have a more passive role in sex because they have to physically open their bodies to let in the male partner. This creates the need for more total relaxation and surrender to the male. Being submissive or playing a submissive role allows women to let go and surrender to the process.

For men who have experienced the pressure of having to be in control over the course of their careers, being submissive can be a temporary relief from the burden of constant responsibility.

Try the next exercise if you haven't explored being submissive or want to learn more about yourself and what it would be like to be in that position.

EXERCISE
Submission Is in Your Mind

Find a place for you and your partner to sit or lie down comfortably for twenty to thirty minutes. Find a pen and paper to answer the following questions. After you are both through, you will move into a dialogue and discuss your answers. Remember that the dialogue allows for intense listening and validation, and is not about agreeing to anything at this time.

Step One
Write down a few sentences that describe what it would be like for you to be submissive in bed. For example: What would happen? What would it look like? Can you describe it? What would you be doing? What would your partner be doing? How? Who would do what?

Step Two
Now write about what it would be like to be dominant in bed, using the questions in Step One.

Step Three
Now decide who will be the sender and who will be the receiver. Senders go first and share their fantasies with their partner. Receivers mirror back what the sender says. Senders share with their partner which fantasy they are the most curious about. The receiver mirrors, validates, and empathizes with the sender.

Step Four
Switch.

Balanced Sexuality

Healthy sexuality is a balance. But for those who suppress their needs, either in the masculine (directive) role or in the feminine (receptive) role, the repressed needs and energy actually grow stronger. We all have both male and female energy, aspects of our personalities and our sexuality that, when in balance, bring a sense of wholeness and peace. Have you ever tried to hold down your feelings? Eventually they come up, and sometimes they sneak up without warning.

The need for balanced sexuality may include a desire to be in both roles, with a preference for one. Perhaps being told what to do takes the pressure off. Being in the submissive role can help you let go of performance pressure, physically and psychologically.

Male or female, acting out a submissive role, surrendering to someone else, can bring a heightened sense of control. Submissives actually have control over the scene. They can relax into the experience, and then go back to their normal way of relating after the role-play is over. They can take back their control and their illusion of power after the session.

Acting out an erotic game by playing with power and control can sometimes create anxiety. Letting go of control by being in sexual submission pushes our edge and increases stress. Pushing our edge forces us to deal with our fears. The stress combined with eroticism forces the body into a heightened state of arousal, releasing a combination of brain chemicals commonly found in people in a "fight or flight state." This stress in the mind creates anxiety and erotic tension at the same time. Overriding this response, and allowing the body to find pleasure in the submissive role, may rewire the brain to live with stress in a different way outside of the scene.

In other words, if in the moment the submissive experiences some panic but then has an orgasm, then the panic becomes linked in the brain with pleasure. When slight sensations of pain are experienced during BDSM play (for example, pinched nipples), then that slight pain becomes connected to pleasure. This confuses the senses and breaks down resistance. When the submissive experiences the confused sensation of being out of control along with erotic pleasure, the pleasure gets linked in the brain. The body holds a memory of the pleasure/pain response it experienced during the BDSM session.

One doesn't need to always act out the BDSM play. Sometimes fantasy can bring us to this place. Going to the pain/pleasure places in the mind can begin to connect pain and pleasure with the areas in ourselves where anxiety lurks.

The Dominant

Dominants in a sexual or erotic game get to feel a heightened sense of control over the world. They are able to experience being powerful, which can increase their sense of self-esteem. Dominants get to be the director. They get to write the script, act the part, and direct the scene. They also have the responsibility of keeping the submissive safe and turned on.

Dominants are responsible for keeping the submissives in their role. Tops develop a keen sense of intuition about their partner's erotic state. Erotic intuition is a heightened level of awareness where all the senses are engaged, including our sixth sense, or intuition. The top's supersensitivity to the bottom's experience engages all of the senses.

Tops get to play the double role of bringing the bottom to the edge of danger and also keeping the bottom safe. They get to inflict discomfort or anxiety on their partner, while also bringing them pleasure.

When dominants can cause pain and pleasure at the same time for their partner, they can become more comfortable and secure in their partnership, outside of the dominant/submissive roles. Dominants actually lose the fear of hurting their partner outside of the BDSM play.

Most men at some time have fears of hurting their partner, emotionally and/or physically. This can create an oversensitive, walking-on-eggshells type of partnership. When dominants feel what its like to play at "hurting" their partner, they begin to understand not only their own power but also the strength and flexibility of their submissive. The range of feelings depends on how fragile they see their partner and how encouraging the submissive is.

If submissives ask to be "disciplined" using pain or control, they are giving permission to their partner that allows for a new freedom of expression. Creating sensation, intense on any level, can be a gift from the top to the bottom.

This freedom and power creates a sense of strength in the world. Knowing that their submissive partner trusts them enough to let them play at being dominant can be a way to feel more committed to the relationship. There is a high level of trust necessary to play the BDSM game. When partners trust each other to stay in the role, and to get each other out when necessary, then all sensation, painful or pleasureable, becomes intense.

The following exercise involves intense role-playing. Find at least ninety minutes or longer where you will not be interrupted. Also, find a safe and comfortable place to act out this role-play. Make sure your phones are off and you will be able to stay in the role for the duration of the exercise.

Set up the room where you will be according to the exercise. If you are the dominant partner for this exercise, be in charge of arranging the furniture, the lighting, and the music in the way that you want it. Take charge of your surroundings, just like you will take charge of your partner.

Tips for Domination Fantasy

Female dominants should dress in black leather or rubber. Use straps and buckles to enhance the outfit, and leave skin and body parts showing. Wear high heels or leather boots. Use a riding crop to "threaten" your partner. "Demand" that he assume positions where you can be in control. Whip him gently, telling him with a forceful voice to get on his knees. Threaten, but do not cause, pain. Have him wear a collar, blindfold, or handcuffs. Tell him what you want him to do to you.

Male dominants should dress up in chaps, a tie, or leather. Tie her hands with scarves or use handcuffs. Talk to her from behind where she can't see you. Blindfold her with a scarf. Keep your clothes on while she strips naked. Tell her how hard you are. Talk dirty. Tell her everything you are planning to do to her before you do it.

Remember that this is erotic play, and it should be fun. If at any time one of you feels uncomfortable, make sure to call a "time out" and ask for a break. Talk about any anxiety or difficulty you are experiencing, and then decide together whether you will continue now or another time. Knowing ahead of time that you can drop the role-play can help both partners trust the BDSM play and relax into it.

Feeling Sensation and Stimulation

All sensation can create a heightened level of arousal. Our physical bodies do not distinguish between different types of arousal. If there is a heightened state of stress, whether it is fear, pain, or pleasure, we react with all our senses.

We become intently focused on the stimulus that is causing us stress. We hear more intensely, we see more clearly, and we smell things we wouldn't normally notice. We observe the passing of time differently. Everything slows down during intense moments of arousal. (Think about what happens during a crisis, such as watching a child run out into the street. The experience of time seems to slow down. Everything feels like it is going in slow motion.)

Any heightened physical state will raise our energy and force us into hyperarousal. This happens when we are scared, stressed, and sexually aroused. The more aroused we are during sex, the slower and more sensual the dance.

Acting out issues around dominance and submission using bondage and control as erotic play can bring up all of our and our partner's "issues." Experimenting with varying levels of sensation can trigger positive and negative psychological baggage from our childhood.

And yet working with pain, control, and power can help heal us from childhood wounds and memories. With a supportive and understanding partner and by talking through feelings, we can heal from memories that may still be influencing us as adults today.

Understanding and Responding to Physical Sensations

This exercise will help you communicate what feels good and give you a language to understand feedback from your partner. It also gives you a way to focus completely on how to give your partner pleasure.

You can use this 1 to 5 number system during sex. If your partner hits areas that feel like a 4 or 5, tell him or her. Feedback is important for great sexual communication.

EXERCISE

Rating the Touch

While sitting comfortably across from one another, senders hold the receiver's arm so that the forearm is face up. Receivers can close their eyes and relax.

Using a scale of 1 to 5—with 1 meaning "I don't like that" and 5 meaning "I love that" (3 would mean okay)—give the sender feedback on the way he touches your forearm. The sender can start with slow, soft touches to the wrist area.

As the sender moves up the arm to a different spot, the receiver gives a 1 to 5 response. The sender changes the type of touch from light scratching to deeper rubbing.

When the receiver gives a higher number response, the sender can continue that pressure and sensation until he finds a touch that results in a 5 response.

Being focused on our partners is like a slow, sensual dance, where you follow their steps, or lead them in the dance, becoming perfectly in tune with their rhythms and their breath. The generosity of being totally present and focused on your partner brings a sense of connection and togetherness.

A Case Example of Control and Light Bondage

Mary and Robert came to therapy to create a deeper and more intense connection. They had been drifting apart as a result of Robert's busy work schedule, and they hadn't had sex in months.

After several sessions they felt reconnected and had made love every weekend for a month. They worked on being able to talk about fantasies, and they had done some exercises at home. One day they came into my office describing a recent sexual experience they had.

Mary described the night before. They had talked about a fantasy that Robert had never shared with her before.

Mary: "He wanted to be tied up."

Robert (smiling): "It was just a fantasy with some light bondage. I always wanted to try it, but never had the nerve to tell Mary about it. I was afraid she would think it was weird, or I was weird."

Mary: "So, anyway, that night, as a surprise, I waited in the bedroom undressed. I was trying to be generous and initiate for once. I was waiting up for Robert to come home. Of course he was late, but that's another story. So he finally comes home and sees me and takes off all his clothes and jumps in bed.

I pulled out some silk scarves that I had hidden under the pillow, and flipped him over, and tied his wrists to the headboard."

I asked her how she was feeling at that point

Mary: "Well, I felt awkward and uncomfortable at first. I am usually the one who waits for Robert to initiate sex. But I wanted to give him his fantasy. He wanted me to be in control. And I wanted to try it for once. So, anyway, he was tied up to the bed. He looked nervous but excited."

I asked Robert how he felt at that point.

Robert: "Oh, I was totally turned on. I had a huge erection and thought it was so cool of Mary to do this for me. But I was slightly embarrassed by the whole thing. Surprisingly, her confidence made me relax. She seemed like she was really into it."

Mary: "Yeah, but then he freaked out."

Robert smirked.

Robert: "Yeah, I did."

I asked what happened.

Mary: "Well, I was on top of Robert, sitting on him, and I bent down to kiss him. That's all I did."

Robert: "Yeah and I freaked."

Mary: "Yeah, he said, and I quote, 'You're freaking me out!' So I got totally angry. I was taking this big chance to try something new and he really hurt my feelings."

Robert: "Yeah, I know, but then she left me there, tied up and walked away!"

Mary laughed.

Mary: "I came back and untied him eventually."

"So what do you think happened, Robert?" I asked.

He described what came up for him. He had experienced an overwhelming feeling of panic once he felt that Mary was in charge and that he had no control. Robert was not as comfortable being *out of control* as he thought he would be. As much as he fantasized about Mary taking initiative and letting her take control, he felt anxious and "freaked out" when she took over.

Mary had felt angry and hurt, not only because she felt rejected, but also because she worried that she had done something wrong. They talked about what control meant to each of them and how it played out in their relationship.

Robert began to talk about his family business, and how his father was overly involved. He talked about how controlling his father was in the business. Robert realized that because of the resentment toward his father, he was anxious when someone else was in control. It was important for Robert to feel like he had power and control over his life.

When Mary realized that the issue of control had more to do with his childhood issues than about her, she softened toward him. They decided that they would try it again, inching Robert closer to his fantasy without making him anxious.

The next night Mary tied one of Robert's wrists to the bedpost, and lay down by his side. Robert experienced his fantasy in a manageable way. He felt more and more that his issues around control were being healed this way. They continued to work together to help Robert with his anxieties.

Robert continued to be the more dominant, directive partner in their sex life, but with Mary's help he was able to realize the other side of his erotic spectrum and push his edge. He felt he was growing as a person and as a sexual partner. Sexually they were able to work through it and begin to heal from their own childhood wounds.

How to Be Sensually Generous

7

"Generous: Characterized by a noble or forbearing spirit: magnanimous, kindly; liberal in giving: open-handed ... ."

—*The Merriam-Webster Dictionary*

Sensual generosity is the desire to give sexually for the pleasure of giving. It's an advanced skill used to channel more sexual energy into a relationship. The bonus of being sensually generous is that generosity begets generosity. The more we give, the more we receive what we want in our relationship.

Being generous toward your partner means allowing your partner to experience the moment without the pressure to reciprocate. Sometimes, sensual generosity means giving yourself over to your lover. However, being willing to give over your body to someone else can feel risky. It may be hard to trust that you won't be hurt or judged when you let someone in, let someone see, and let someone touch. Allowing yourself to feel vulnerable is an act of generosity toward the other person.

Generosity also means being open and willing to hear and experience the other person's fantasies—and possibly participating in those fantasies. It necessitates empathizing with someone else's feelings and understanding how our behavior affects our partner. Generosity requires you to have insight into your own issues and where they come from, and then have the generosity to change, sometimes in ways you would prefer not to.

In other words, our capacity to give to our partner and expect nothing in return can be limited, depending on how comfortable we are with generosity.

Most of us would like to think that we are generous and giving people, especially in bed, and yet we may wonder whether what happens in bed feels "fair" sometimes.

Allowing yourself to feel vulnerable
is an act of generosity toward the other person.

Keeping score about who gives more and who takes more detracts from a relationship. Partners who fear and worry that they won't get their needs met, perhaps because of past experiences, may hold back their generosity, hoping that they will get the time and attention they have long desired. On the other hand, partners who feel they always give—like a martyr—may hold back, hoping that this will get them the love and the sex they want.

It actually works the other way around. The more we give, the more responsive our partner becomes, and the more we can receive.

Our "Imago," or the "image" of the person we seek out in relationships, is a conglomeration of character traits that we hope will give us what we long for. We can end up disappointed and frustrated when our partners don't act like we want them to. It can be hard to give without the fear that we won't receive.

George and Martine—When Giving Means More

The beauty of choosing our Imago match is that by giving our partners what they need, we actually grow into the partner we need to become. For example, George and Martine came to my office for couples counseling because Martine felt neglected and ignored by George.

Martine came from a loving family, but had felt ignored by her father because he traveled often for work. She had chosen George as a partner because she saw that George focused on her needs. He was a generous sexual partner, always trying to please her in bed. But she wanted more. She felt invisible with him. He also felt that she withheld sex from him as punishment if he didn't give her enough attention. He wanted her to be more assertive in bed and to sometimes take charge. Martine said she wasn't in the mood for sex when she didn't feel connected to George.

Martine's growth gift in her relationship was to move toward what George wanted from her. He wanted her to take charge in bed. He felt her need to be seen would be met as a result.

Martine was able to push her growth edge. She was able to move into the area where George wanted her to grow and not be focused on how she wanted George to change. She was able to take the risk and initiate sex several times, being more assertive in bed. She pushed herself to grow in the way that George needed, and she put her own needs aside.

When she did this, she realized that she was actually getting more of what she wanted from George: attention and appreciation. She felt special and cherished by George, which is what she had needed as a child. Her growth was moving her into the areas where she most needed healing. And it was through her sexual generosity with George that his need to feel loved from Martine was fulfilled.

Getting Past "Not Being in the Mood"

Sometimes giving sex to our partners when we don't want to can feel like a chore. But caring for them—and being sexually generous—sometimes means we do things we don't want to do because we know it will bring pleasure to our partner.

When you aren't in the mood for sex, there are still things you can do for your partner that can help him feel pleasure. Being sensually generous might mean reaching out and touching your partner, even if you don't want to make love or have intercourse.

Sometimes pushing yourself to have a piece of lovemaking, but not the whole pie, can satisfy both of you. Giving or receiving manual stimulation—sometimes all the way to orgasm—is one example. Another is just experiencing the pleasure of touching your partner and enjoying the moment.

Having quick sex to satisfy your partner's needs can be a way to show generosity and stay connected, even when you are not in the mood to have a long lovemaking session.

In addition, mutual masturbation is something that can satisfy both of you, and it serves a dual purpose. When we masturbate in front of our partners, they learn what feels good by watching our technique. They see what we do to bring ourselves to orgasm and can use this information at another time to connect more deeply with our pleasure. It can also be a turn-on for them to watch us touch ourselves.

As noted previously, one way to be more interested in lovemaking is to consciously set the stage for sex by making a date night. It can also be a reminder that taking the time for sex is a priority in the relationship.

EXERCISE
Creating Rituals around Sex

Lighting candles, giving massages, and creating other such rituals around lovemaking can increase the mood. A ritual is something we do with concentrated mindfulness, to create an "occasion" for sex.

In this exercise, decide who will be the sender and the receiver. The receiver's job is to relax and receive pleasure, and the sender's job is to make the experience as sensual as possible. Without expectation of anything in return, experience the joy that being generous can bring you, as the sender, as you feel your partner's receptivity and pleasure.

Plan a night for sex. Make sure that your partner is available and that you have ample, uninterrupted time. You should both have the opportunity to go directly to sleep when you are through. Make sure the room is warm and lit with candles or low lighting. Pull the drapes, put on sexy music, and create scents with rose petals, fragrant candles, or incense.

Take a long, hot bath with fragrant bath oil.

Put soft sheets on the bed. Add extra pillows for comfort and sensuality. Have a lubricant and massage oils handy by the bed. Choose sexy lingerie or underwear that has texture and softness to it.

When your partner comes into the room touch him slowly, gently pulling him into the mood and allowing him to adjust to a slower, more sensual tempo.

Step One

Give your partner the gift of a full body, sensual massage. Reassure your partner that there are no strings attached to the massage. Give the massage freely, without expectation that sex will happen as a result or that there will be reciprocation of the massage.

Begin by spreading the massage oil on your partner's back and then out to the extremities. Make sure you use enough pressure so that your partner feels your fingers in the muscles. Ask your partner whether he or she would like softer or harder strokes. Try not to ask, "Is it okay?" Instead, be specific, always offering your partner the chance to direct you to make it harder or softer.

Then let your partner relax into the massage without talking. Use broad hand strokes and simple massaging motions with your palms.

Step Two

Now try squeezing different body parts with the flats of your hands. Hold muscles or body parts gently, letting the warmth from your hands relax your partner's muscles.

Step Three

Now scratch gently with your fingertips and nails. Trace the outline of your partner's body with your hand, from the base of the neck to the perineum. Part his or her buttocks softly, taking each one in hand and stroking deeply. Rub the insides of the thighs with long, deep strokes upward, bringing energy to the genitals.

Remember to breathe while you massage. The receiver can let out any sighs or moans or signs of appreciation for the experience.

Step Four

Now speak softly about how much you appreciate your partner's body. You could whisper things like, "Your skin is so soft," "Your shoulders are so strong," or "I love your thighs." If your partner tries to talk or thank you for the compliment, respond by gently whispering "shh."

Step Five

Continue until your partner falls asleep or the massage naturally moves into lovemaking.

Sharing One Another

We need to be open to sharing ourselves with another person, which is what creates true intimacy and connection. Letting someone else "in" emotionally can sometimes be harder than letting someone "in" to your body.

The next exercise will allow you to experience the connection with your partner in a deep and nonverbal way. Our eyes are the windows to our soul, and the left eye, in Tantric yoga, is considered the receptive eye. Gazing into your lover's left eye helps you focus on that person and look deeply into the true self. Receiving your partner's gaze can be a way to open up and allow him or her into your intimate space.

For this exercise, you will need a warm room, with no distractions. Make sure there is quiet or soft music playing in the background. Carve out uninterrupted time for yourselves, and set up the room for a full sensual experience. Put fresh flowers by the bed, turn down the lights (but not to total darkness), and put down soft blankets to sit on.

EXERCISE
Intimacy or "In-To-Me-See"

This is an exercise you do sitting up and facing each other. Sit as close together as possible—one classic way to sit is with the female partner on top of the legs of the male partner, with her legs wrapped around behind him. Both of you are sitting on your buttocks, but your legs form a cocoon that surrounds the both of you. This way you can be in close physical contact, and you will be more likely to feel your partner's belly when he or she breathes.

If this is not physically comfortable, sit as close as possible with legs overlapping, and find a position that you can maintain for several moments. Remember you can always shift around throughout the exercise if you feel uncomfortable.

Step One

Relax your shoulders. Breathe deeply and into your belly. As you breathe, try to register your partner's breathing. Notice when your partner inhales and exhales. See whether you can coordinate your breathing so that you both breathe together, at the same time.

Step Two

Gaze directly into your partner's left eye; the left eye is the receptive eye. See whether, with each breath, you can welcome your partner nonverbally into your body. Breathe your partner in as you gaze into his or her left eye.

Keep the breathing up for at least fifty breaths. You don't need to count out loud, but try to let yourself truly relax into the breathing.

Step Three

When you are ready to stop, take a final deep, cleansing breath and exhale with an audible sigh. Smile at your partner.

Step Four

Take a last deep breath in and ask your partner whether now is a good time to share. Using the Imago method of mirroring, share with your partner what it felt like to breathe together. Try to talk about any emotions that came up for you, including feelings of love, sadness, happiness, and anger.

This might sound like the following:

Sender: "When I was breathing with you, I felt deeply connected to you."

Receiver: "When you were breathing with me, you felt deeply connected to me."

Sender: "Yes, and I experienced many emotions. I felt deep love for you, and I also felt some sadness."

Receiver: "So you felt deep love for me and also some sadness."

Sender: "Yes, I felt sadness because I have missed you these past few weeks. But then I felt joy that I have you here now and that I love being with you."

Receiver: "So you felt sadness because you have missed me these past few weeks, but then you felt joy that I am here now and that you love being with me. Did I get that? Is there more?"

(continued on page 158)

(continued)

Step Five
Switch.

Step Six
When you are done mirroring one another, share one thing with each other that you appreciated about this intimacy exercise. For example:

Sender: "One thing I really appreciated about this exercise with you is how intimate and connected it felt."

Receiver: "So one thing you really appreciated about this exercise with me is how intimate and connected you felt."

Step Seven
If now is a good time to make love, you may find yourself naturally moving into pleasing each other. Or you may drift off to sleep in each other's arms.

How "Faking It" Hurts a Relationship

Sometimes generosity means being receptive to pleasure. Being blocked from receiving pleasure can be caused by many things—guilt around sexuality, poor body image, low self-esteem, or an inability to express our feelings. All of these things are important to recognize so that we can change how we receive pleasure, not just for us, but for our partners!

Our feelings about ourselves can interfere with our capacity to receive pleasure. Low self-esteem, for example, is expressed sometimes in the fear that "if you really knew me you wouldn't like me." Low self-esteem prevents us from letting our partners get close to us, because we fear that they won't like what they see.

One of the ways to improve self-esteem is by recognizing the parts of ourselves that our partner appreciates. Sometimes asking for those appreciations from our partner can help reinforce our positive traits. Yet, finding this self-confidence in ourselves is important. Our partners will find us infinitely more desirable and interesting if we believe the positive things about ourselves—self-assurance and confidence are very attractive in a partner.

Self-esteem is sometimes affected by how we feel about our bodies. Body image issues are chronic in our society. For women, the perceived failure to uphold the ideal body type personified by models and advertising images can create a feeling of dissatisfaction and even embarrassment about their body.

Only a small percentage of women will ever uphold the body type of a fashion model. And yet the majority of women compare themselves to this standard. Knowing that your body is unique and beautiful because of its size and shape helps improve body image distortions.

For men, body image is often tied up with performance. Men perceive themselves as being less than or better than, depending on their body shape and penis size. Penis size is not a direct correlation with sexual satisfaction in women. When men understand how to be sensual and sexually generous, they can heal from the anxiety around whether their penis is large enough.

Interestingly, when we care about our partners and are attracted to them, we focus on the areas we like and appreciate. This is part of sexual attraction. Most of the time, our partners focus on the parts of our bodies they adore and cherish. And yet the fear that we are unattractive prevents us from feeling comfortable in our bodies when we make love.

It is important to share these feelings with our partners. If you share your fears and insecurities with your partner, he or she will be less likely to take it personally when you hold back during sex. If you keep your clothes on, keep the lights off, or hide yourself in general, your partner may perceive this behavior as a wall between the two of you, and your partner might take it personally.

Being generous means reassuring your partner that your self-protection is not about him or her. Sharing your insecurity can reassure your partner and also help you to work on your own self-image.

Allowing Yourself Pleasure with Your Partner

It can be hard to receive reassurance from your partner. It can also be hard to receive pleasure because of it. Blocking pleasure from your relationship keeps the partnership from getting to the next level of intimacy and connection.

Although many women fake orgasms, they need to recognize that this is not a generous act.

Consider this example. A couple came into my office for sex and relationship counseling and described their relationship as "full of stress and without pleasure." Both partners wanted their partnership to be a place where they felt comfortable and secure, as well as alive and passionate.

The couple described their love life as "boring" and not particularly satisfying to either of them. When I asked them how often they had sex, they said they made love several times a week. I asked whether the female partner had orgasms.

"Not when we have sex," she said. "I can give myself an orgasm when I am alone, if I do it myself. But with him, I really can't come. And I don't think it's a big deal. I can have sex without an orgasm; it's fine."

Her partner, when asked, said he loved to give a woman an orgasm. He insisted he was "totally into it." He said he had been able to give women orgasms in the past without difficulty. I asked how he did that, and he said that his partners had always described to him exactly what they liked and wanted. He went further to describe his feelings about giving a woman an orgasm. He said he "got off on it."

I wondered, how many men feel the same way? When I surveyed the men in my practice and talked to male friends, each one told me that his number one priority during sex was to give his partner an orgasm! I explored this further and realized that men feel successful, powerful, and turned on when their partner reaches orgasm.

Talking to the couple in my office, I empathized with the woman and validated her feelings. I also told her that making sure she had an orgasm was not really about her, but about him. If she were to be generous enough to teach her partner what she needed to climax during sex, she would be giving him an incredible gift! The gift for men is to help them feel powerful in the relationship.

She said she had always felt that her orgasm was "not necessary" and didn't want to "burden" her partner with her needs. He disagreed with her and said her orgasm was "very" necessary, not just for her, but also for him! (This is illustrated later in this chapter with Don and Julie.)

Leading the Way

Generosity of spirit—giving to the other—and generosity with one's own body sometimes mean letting someone else experience the landscape of the self.

Although many women fake orgasms, they need to recognize that this is not a generous act. It is actually a setup for their partners to misunderstand their sexual needs. It prevents their partner from fully understanding what it means to give pleasure. This deprives them of the opportunity to be generous.

Our partners have no way of understanding how our bodies work unless we tell them. Even when two women are in a sexual relationship, they need to communicate how to stimulate each other. All bodies are different and can have slight variations in the ways that they respond to stimulation.

We make assumptions in relationships that if our partners really loved us they would be able to read our minds. Actually, they can't understand what our sexual needs are unless we tell them! And most of us don't come with instructions, so how can our partners know what works unless we teach them?

The following exercise will help women communicate with their partners about what they desire sexually. It is a direct and easy way to help women find a language to describe their sexual needs. Using this exercise can help decrease the fear that sometimes prevents women from being verbal about what they like in bed.

With this language, and with the Imago dialogue, women can learn to express their deepest sexual desires, and also teach their partners exactly what they need in order to reach orgasm.

To get the sex you really want, you have to help your partner know what that means. Remember that when we use the Imago language we can express our feelings and be heard. Our partner can listen in an active and direct way. This takes away the feeling of being judged for our needs and desires.

EXERCISE
Clitoral Clock

To do this exercise, you will need a quiet place where you will not be interrupted for at least sixty minutes. Set up the room (preferably with a bed) so that both of you will be warm, relaxed, and comfortable. Find soft music, fresh flowers, incense, or candles for the room. Make sure your phones are off and that there is sufficient light to see, but that the room is softly lit.

For the following exercise you will also need a lubricant. Any water-based lubricant will work, or use vegetable-based massage oils. (Please note that any scents or warming additive in personal lubricants can cause urinary tract infections and should be avoided.)

Make sure that as the sender your hands are clean and your nails filed or cut short. Keep in mind that the female vulva, including the clitoris, is tender and delicate but can withstand a lot of pressure to bring to orgasm.

The female partner, the receiver, can disrobe and lay in a comfortable place on the bed. Make sure the position is one that is comfortable for a long period of time, and gives access to the sender to touch and see the genitals.

Receivers should let themselves be in a receptive mode. Take deep breaths and allow your body to relax. Feel the opening in yourself as you spread your legs. Make eye contact with the sender and ask for any kiss, touch, or holding that you need before you begin.

Senders should be in a position to see and touch the receiver's vulva. Check with the receiver to make sure she is comfortable and whether she needs anything before you begin. Always warm up your hands before touching naked skin by rubbing your hands together rapidly or blowing warm air into your palms.

Step One
Start by touching the receiver's legs, rubbing your hands over her calves and over the knees and up onto the inner thighs. As you feel your partner relax, open the lubricant and spread it on your fingers as well as her vulva, paying particular attention to the clitoral area.

Using lots of lubricant, warm up your partner's clitoris and vagina with soft stroking and gentle rubbing. Then, imagine the clitoris as a clock, with twelve o'clock being the top portion of the clitoris closest to the belly. Using a well-lubricated finger or two, move clockwise in a small circular motion from the twelve o'clock to one o'clock position and around the clitoris, back to the twelve o'clock position. Do this slowly and repeat it several times.

Step Two

Now have your partner comment on each "time" position and tell you on a scale of 1 to 5 how that position feels to be stimulated and how intense the feeling is. Here, 1 means nonresponsive or uncomfortable, 2 is slightly pleasurable, 3 means "okay, starting to feel good," 4 is wonderful, and 5 is the best and will create an orgasm if it is continued. If you are the sender, tell your partner what time position she is in and wait for a response. This may sound like:

Sender: "This is one o'clock. How does that feel?"

Receiver: "Oh, that's a 4!"

Continue around the clitoris to each time, telling your partner where you are and asking how it feels for her on a scale of 1 to 5.

Step Three

Continue the slow circular motion using different strokes and pressures, and explore other areas of the vulva, always asking the receiver for feedback, using the 1 to 5 scale.

Step Four

Continue until you can bring your partner to orgasm. Keep in mind that even if your partner is at a 5, you may need to back down occasionally to a 3 or 4 level of stimulation. Bringing her back up and then back down can prolong the pleasure and make the orgasm more intense.

Also note that stimulation to orgasm can take anywhere from eight to thirty minutes for women.

The Scorekeeping Sabotage

In relationships we might find ourselves using sex as a way to keep score. We might add up the times we initiate sex, or we might keep track of how often we are the givers. Perhaps we become supersensitive to how often we are the instigators of creative sex, which our partner receives grudgingly and, many times, unwillingly.

Scorekeeping in our sexual relationships can also be a result of keeping score of who does the most household chores, or how often our partner makes an effort to connect with us. When sex is used as a way to even the score, our relationships suffer. Partnerships are not always equal.

Many times I meet with couples in my office and the session turns into a discussion of "who gave who what." One example might be a woman who comes into my office and resents her partner because he often expresses his desire for more oral sex. "He talks ad nauseum about blow jobs," she says. "That's all he wants. And yet, does he give me oral sex as much as I want it?"

She is keeping track of who gave whom oral sex, and how many times. She also wants to know:

"Do I really have to do it, and how come that's all he wants, and when do my needs come first, and why should I do that for him?"

What she really wants to know is: "How can I give him a blow job when I am so mad at him?"

What he really wants to know is: "How can we ever get over all this stuff so we can finally have sex?"

If women need emotional intimacy to be in the mood for sex, men need sex to feel intimate emotionally. What happens when there is a standoff? Eventually no one is intimate and no one is having sex!

If your resentments are getting in the way, here is an exercise to help work through them so that you both can have the sex you want.

EXERCISE
Locking Up Resentment

Sometimes our resentment can get in the way of being a sexually generous partner. If we use this containment exercise and learn new ways to communicate our resentment using the Imago techniques, we can get past our resistance and allow our sensual generosity to create a more connected partnership.

Step One

Imagine an antique trunk on a shelf in your closet. The trunk has a beautiful old padlock and brass straps around it. Visualize yourself putting all your resentment and frustrations in the trunk. In your mind, lock the trunk. Notice whether you feel more in the mood to have sex with your partner.

If not, explore whether there are other resentments that you might not have locked away. If so, add them to the trunk.

Step Two

Now put the trunk back on the shelf. Close the closet door in your imagination. Walk away!

You can take down the trunk anytime and feel free to pull out the resentments later. When you are ready to have a dialogue with your partner about your resentments, you can use the Imago techniques to communicate your feelings, but notice whether now, in this moment, you can let go of them.

Step Three

Tell your partner three things you appreciated about him or her when you first met. Have your partner mirror back everything you say.

Step Four

Now have your partner tell you three things he or she appreciated about you when you first met. Mirror everything back.

Notice whether you feel more connected. Take note: are you open to giving or receiving sexual pleasure in this moment? If not, appreciate the moment of connection with your partner.

Giving Up Control

In addition to holding on to resentments, we can also have difficulty being generous because we want to remain in control. Control issues keep us from letting go and moving toward our partners and giving them what they ask for.

The following case example illustrates how control plays into our sexual relationships and gives clear ideas about letting go and moving toward what our partner wants from us. In this way, we grow as individuals.

Melissa and Jason came into my office complaining of "difficulty" in their marriage. The sex was acceptable, but not what either of them really wanted. They had no experience talking about what they needed, and did not understand the language necessary to talk about erotic needs. They both wanted to learn how to reconnect.

One afternoon in their session together, Jason appeared withdrawn. Melissa was on the edge of her seat and looked tense and angry. Her fists were clenched and she crossed her arms over her chest.

Jason: "I think Melissa is withholding sex." He looked angry and hurt. His face was set in a grimace and he avoided making eye contact.

Melissa: "All Jason wants is oral sex! All he wants is a blow job, and he wants it the same way every time."

I asked Melissa what she wanted.

Melissa: "I want to feel connected to Jason. When I give him oral sex I feel disconnected and distant from him. It also hurts my jaw and I get cramped from the same motion over and over."

Jason: "So, Melissa, what you are saying is that you want to feel connected to me, and that giving oral sex makes you feel disconnected and it hurts your jaw."

Jason mirrored what she said, without offering a solution. Sometimes therapists will change the subject and instead of focusing on the sexual issues they will try to shift the focus to the emotional distance in the relationship. Helping a couple talk about sex can be a quicker way in to the relationship. To make some concrete changes in the relationship, why not go straight for the issue that is presenting?

If things change in the sexual relationship, the rest of the relationship can change. It can take many weeks of therapy to change a behavior like "taking out the garbage." And yet, when couples leave a session promising to take out the garbage, they come back a week later in the same pain and frustration they were in when they left. When changes are made in their sexual partnership, real intimacy and connection happens. So I asked Jason to continue mirroring the sexual content of what Melissa was saying.

Jason: "And so what you are saying is that you feel like all I want is a blow job and I want it the same way every time."

Melissa: "Yes, it's boring down there by myself! Nothing is happening for me and you just go into some trance and stop talking to me."

I asked Jason whether there were ways he could stay engaged with Melissa during oral sex.

Jason: "Sometimes oral sex is great for going into a trance. And sometimes, to be honest, I just want to come, and get a release. But if I know she hates doing it, I can't relax, and then it takes me longer to come."

I asked Jason to describe in detail what she did that felt good. Melissa mirrored everything he said. His appreciation of her softened her anxiety.

She relaxed into the session, and even smiled as he described the details of what she did with her tongue that brought him intense pleasure.

Melissa: "Thank you, Jason. I really do want to make you feel good if I can. But I am so lonely down there by myself!"

Jason mirrored Melissa and asked her what she needed. They came up with several ways he could make physical contact with her while she was giving him oral sex.

They agreed to try several things. He would put his hands in her hair and touch her shoulders while she was giving him oral sex. This would help her feel connected to him during the sexual act. This would also give him more of a sense of control, and possibly help him ejaculate sooner during oral sex, which they both identified as a desire that they shared.

Jason also decided that he would try to be more verbal during oral sex. He would talk to her as she was doing it, and tell her exactly what he liked about what she was doing. He would use phrases like, "That feels great when you lick me" or "I love when you suck hard like that."

During this dialogue in the office, as they mirrored back and forth, Melissa made more eye contact with Jason and he gazed into her eyes and held her hands. Their bodies were relaxed, and they were no longer angry or frustrated with each other. Melissa even described that she felt aroused by the conversation, and that it "turned her on" to hear what Jason wanted during a blow job.

The final part of the dialogue was about Melissa's desire to feel aroused while she was giving Jason oral sex.

Melissa: "I think I would feel more connected to you, and to the whole experience, if I was turned on. I just can't get into it sometimes."

Jason: "Can you keep eye contact with me during a blow job?"

Although that seemed difficult for both of them, she agreed to try. Jason also brought up another fun option.

Jason: "Melissa, can you use a vibrator to stimulate yourself while you give me a blow job? I would love to watch that while you are giving me head!"

He said he would feel more engaged with her in this way as well, watching what she was doing.

I suggested they have oral sex in small doses throughout the week, without bringing Jason to climax. This would increase Melissa's comfort level and decrease her resentment around being made to "get him off all the time." It would also help her to relax her muscles and learn ways to give oral sex that would not hurt her jaw. Most pain during oral sex can be alleviated when the jaw is relaxed.

Melissa also liked the idea of moving her hand on his penis while the head was in her mouth. She agreed to try the vibrator while she was giving him oral sex, and said she would be happier starting in small sessions, perhaps building up to longer periods as they practiced more of the connecting exercise.

During the dialogue the couple sat across from each other, facing each other and made eye contact. Melissa relaxed, sat back in her chair, and smiled at Jason. They made physical contact several times by holding hands, and laughed together when they were feeling shy.

The following week Jason and Melissa reported an amazing difference not only in their sexual relationship, which actually had not changed all that dramatically, but also in their capacity to talk about what was happening between them.

Jason: "Hey, I figured if we could talk about blow jobs for an hour we can pretty much talk about anything now!"

Melissa said she felt heard and understood, and no longer felt resentful. She said Jason had talked to her about how important it was for him to have these new experiences with her. She was more attached to him and felt more empathetic to his needs.

EXERCISE
Bonding over Oral Sex

The following exercise illustrates ways to stay connected to your partner, and helps with some of the resistance that you may feel when your partner wants something that feels uncomfortable for you.

During oral sex, first make eye contact. Then touch the giver's hair. Use words that describe how you are feeling in every moment. Focus on the experience, or the journey, and try to stay in the moment. Focusing on bringing your partner to orgasm can take away from the feelings of connection in the present. This is not a race to the end zone; it is an experience that you are having as a couple, to be enjoyed by both of you.

Sharing Erotic Needs with Each Other

Men and women share similar erotic needs. They also have specific needs that are determined by their gender. Some of the needs that both men and women desire include safety, trust, connection, intensity, challenge, fantasy, fear, thrill, comfort, and passion. Most of us have these needs at some level.

However, men and women also have erotic needs that are specific not only to their gender, but also to them as individuals. We have erotic tendencies that are special to us as a result of the way we grew up, how we were socialized, and how our own physical anatomy works.

EXERCISE
Sharing Our Sexual Needs

This exercise is a way to get to know your partner and compare your needs. Go down the list below and number each item according to how important this need is for you, rating it from 1 (not so important) to 10 (very important).

- Safety
- Trust
- Connection
- Intensity
- Challenge
- Fantasy
- Fear
- Thrill
- Comfort
- Passion

Have your partner do the same. Now compare lists. What do you notice about yourself and your needs? How do they compare with your partner's needs?

When Gender Makes the Difference

Sometimes we assume that because we need something, our partners should have the same need. We assume that they should know what we want because, hey, don't they want the same thing? The more we experience the erotic needs of our partners as different from our own, the more we can begin to understand who they are.

Differentiation is an advanced-level skill, but one that, when mastered, allows us some space in our relationship. And it is in this space that the longing, or the desire for another, happens. We begin to crave connection when we feel separate. This draws us to our partners and creates more intensity in the sexual relationship.

If we are totally merged with our partners, thinking they are the same as us, and want the same things and think the same way, then there is no space between us and we become overly familiar with that partner. Even though most of this is what we call projection—where we attribute certain qualities to another that are really about ourselves—we are often unaware that we do it.

We still look at our partners as extensions of ourselves, and it takes work and maturity to see them as separate people with their own unique thoughts and needs. If we can begin to see our partners that way, we can begin to understand some of their fantasies and needs, but in a new way. Now perhaps they make sense to us, and perhaps we can even fulfill those fantasies if we understand that they are not about what we want, but what our partner wants.

Men's Sexual Needs

Keeping in mind that we are all unique, most men have the following erotic needs, which are explained in detail below:

1. Physical connection. Men need to have a physical connection with their partner to feel confident and secure. Sex, to men, is an important way to find emotional security. The physicality of the erotic bond helps men feel open to communicating and talking about their feelings. Having someone to hold and touch is a powerful way for men to relate.

Direct genital contact is important for men as well. Sometimes taking our time and teasing before we get to a man's penis or scrotum is wonderful, but men need to have direct contact in the places that feel the best. Their lead time is shorter than a woman's and they crave a direct, confident touch in the places that arouse them.

2. Generosity or pleasing a partner. Men generally agree on one thing: that pleasing their partner is one of their priorities. Making a woman happy in bed, giving her an orgasm, and being sure she is enjoying the erotic connection is so important to men that when they don't feel like they are pleasing their partner they can become depressed and discouraged. See the sidebar on page 172.

3. Appreciation. Because men have spent their whole lives being recognized for what they do and not for who they are, many perceive their actions to be their most important contribution to the world.

Often the question people ask a man when they first meet is "What do you do?" The implication is that what they *do* is the most important aspect of who they *are*. This is not as true for women. Girls don't necessarily have to perform to get recognition. There is certainly pressure on girls to do well in school, and there is increased competition to get into college, which provokes more ambitious and creative forces in girls. Often, however, girls are still recognized and judged for their looks, regardless of their accomplishments.

Boys, on the other hand, are recognized for how they behave: the grades they get, the sports they play, and how they act. As adults, men still focus on their accomplishments, at least until they get older and begin to doubt their whole direction in life, which is the midlife awakening so often called the "midlife crisis."

Midlife *awakening* happens when men reach a developmental age where they have experienced some success in their lives, and they begin to realize that who they *are* does not necessarily translate into what they *do*. Perhaps they have worked hard all their lives to provide for a family or to pursue monetary or social success.

He Needs You to Come

Don and June came to my office because of June's inability to have an orgasm.

"It doesn't really matter to me if I have an orgasm with Don," June said. "I can do it when I am alone and masturbating, so I know I am capable of having one. But with Don, it's fine if we just make love and I don't come. It doesn't honestly matter to me." Don looked upset, and I asked him how he felt about it.

"Well, it matters to me," he said. "I don't enjoy sex with June if I know she won't have an orgasm."

I assured June that it is certainly enjoyable to have sex with someone you care about, knowing that he is enjoying himself, and that its not always necessary for women to have an orgasm every time. It's not always necessary for men to have an orgasm every time either! Yet, even though she claimed that she didn't need to orgasm during sex with Don, it was very important for Don. She needed to work on having an orgasm with him, not for her, but for him! And the way to do that was to teach Don how she made herself come.

Teaching your partner how to give you an orgasm is not just about your own pleasure; it also allows your partner to experience your generosity. Both partners can do this, one at a time, during one session, or in two separate sessions. Each partner should go slowly so the other can watch you and see exactly what you are doing and where you are touching yourself. Show your partner how you touch yourself to reach orgasm.

If you feel up to it, describe in detail what you are doing as you masturbate. Tell your partner about your preferences. You might say something like, "I love touching my clit on the bottom softly at first and then I go around it slowly, but with more pressure, like this." After you've reached orgasm, switch with your partner and watch him masturbate as he describes exactly what he does to ejaculate.

When you are through, you may find that you feel slightly embarrassed or self-conscious. You will also feel closer and more intimate with your partner. Now is the time to have a quiet dialogue, perhaps lying next to one another.

Midlife awakening happens when men reach a developmental age that allows them to experience success in their lives, and they have come to a place in life when they realize that who they are does not necessarily translate into what they do.

By midlife, most men begin to realize and wake up to the fact that they have never truly been able to "feel," that is, they have not been encouraged to express their emotional side but have had to repress their feelings to get by in the world. By midlife they discover that they have a wealth of emotions and a new sensitivity to the world where they crave feeling. These men sometimes gravitate toward women (or cars) that make them feel something. Some men get overwhelmed by their emotions, and others become more giving and spiritual.

Many men at midlife become better lovers because they begin to grow out of the intense self-focus and pressure to perform. They seek things in life that give them deeper satisfaction and meaning. As they age, they work harder to be in the moment.

The focus on men's actions influences their erotic needs. They need to be appreciated for their actions and their accomplishments. They want to be recognized for what they do—a need they have had since early childhood.

Whether it means feeling appreciated for bringing out the garbage or for giving their partner an orgasm, they need the feedback in an appreciative way.

Anything that a woman says to a man that is about "not doing" enough will be perceived as criticism. Male sensitivity to appreciation is due to a lifelong need to earn the affirmation around how they are "doing."

Appreciation is something that both men and women need, but men complain more about not getting it. When men complain about their partners, they say things like, "No matter what I do it's never enough" or "She doesn't appreciate all the things I do for her." In their minds, they work at pleasing their partner through their actions. Sometimes those actions may not be appreciated by their partner, since women don't recognize the need to be rewarded for all that they do.

You can work on appreciating your partner by telling him three things you appreciate about him while you are in bed with him. Whisper in his ear things you like that he is doing to you, such as "I love when you tease my nipples like that" or "I love the way your penis feels inside me."

Use explicit words. Don't expect anything in return.

Tell him afterward three things you liked about how he made love to you. Top it off with a kiss. Notice how your partner responds. Tell him what you notice. It might sound like, "You are so cute when I tell you these things—you blush right down to your toes!" or "Your smile is beautiful right now."

4. Action. Because men have been socialized to act, they need to make things happen. Male energy moves things to the next level, to the conclusion, to the end zone. In our culture, sex is often about getting to the finish line, moving things to ejaculation, which is the ultimate destination.

This need to move things to the next place also explains why men take women's flirtation as a sign that the woman is interested in them and that they want to take the relationship to a sexual level. The male need for action is what makes men have a tendency to be more directive and more dominant in relationships and in bed.

5. Languages of love. We all experience love differently. Because of the way we grew up and what we learned about love, we have needs that may not be the same as those of our partners.

Some people experience being loved and giving love in the same way. In his book, *Five Love Languages*, author Gary Chapman describes different ways that we all show and receive love. The five love languages are sex, praise, acts of service, gifts, and time.

Our languages of love are important to understand when we talk about sex and erotic needs. If our partner's language of love is time, then perhaps being in bed for long stretches of time and spending time talking about sex would make that person feel loved. If your partner's language of love is gifts, then small tokens that express thoughtfulness would go a long way toward softening the relationship. Books about sex, lingerie, massage oils, candles—all of these gifts can help your partner feel loved while at the same time improving the atmosphere in your bedroom!

Acts of service include things like keeping the house clean, shopping, building bookcases, and running errands. Doing things for our partners to make their life easier is an example of the love language of acts of service. Praise includes being verbal about things you appreciate about your partner. Sex and affection can be a way to experience love and to show love.

The following case describes ways that we love each other, and how we experience differences between us.

Speaking Different Languages of Love

Tina and Tom came into therapy because they felt the distance in their relationship was growing and they had serious questions about their ability to stay married. After twenty-seven years they wanted to stay committed to each other, but both felt unappreciated and unloved.

Tina: "I stay in the kitchen until late at night, hoping Tom will come down and help me clean up. If he would just do the dishes once in a while, I would be happy to have sex with him."

Tom: "Well, at night I am upstairs in our bed waiting for her to come up and make love. If she really loved me, we would be having sex more often. But she spends all her time futzing around the kitchen and by the time she comes up I'm asleep."

Tina's language of love is acts of service. For her, what Tom does for her to help out shows her that he loves her. She grew up in a family where her father mowed the lawn, built bookshelves, and took her mother shopping. She experienced love as an expression of what people did for her. She felt loved when Tom would unpack the groceries from the car for her.

(continued on page 176)

Speaking Different Languages of Love

(continued)

Tom's language of love is sex and physical affection. He grew up without any physical contact from his parents. Spending most of his life in an orphanage, he was not adopted until he was twelve, and his adopted family was not affectionate. He never played full contact sports, nor did he have a girlfriend until he was twenty-four. He craved physical contact, and he experienced sex and affection as healing. He felt loved when Tina crawled into bed next to him and he would sleep curled up behind her like spoons in a drawer.

Once Tom and Tina understood each other's language of love, they were able to love one another in the way that each needed to be loved. They now saw how each of them had been trying to show love to the other, but in a language the other did not understand or appreciate. The gestures were lost on each of them. When they began to see how the other person experienced that as rejection and abandonment, they were able to change things in the relationship.

Several months later, Tina reported that Tom had installed a new dishwasher for her and was helping her load it every night. They would go to bed together at the same time every night, and most nights Tina would express her appreciation for Tom's efforts and snuggle up to him in bed. Many times that would turn into sex. Tom reported feeling more connected to Tina and became more willing to love her in the ways she needed. Tina understood Tom's needs and was happy to help him feel loved and secure, once she understood how to do that!

Female Sexual Needs

In contrast to men, women have different emotional, physical, and erotic needs. Their sexual needs include the following:

1. Physical affection. For women, physical affection guarantees their security in the relationship. Touch is a way of "checking in" for women. Knowing that her partner is there, and occasionally reaching out to connect in a loving way, helps the female partner feel safe. The need to be acknowledged, to feel like "he knows I am here" is a big one.

When women complain about men, they often say things like, "He doesn't even know I'm here" or "I don't feel like he's present." Feeling physical affection reaffirms for women that their partner is indeed "there" and still cares for them.

2. Long lead time. Women have different needs from men when it comes to foreplay. Women's arousal levels are different, and they need to reach several plateaus before they reach orgasm. These plateaus are the levels of physical arousal that make sex more interesting in the moment. Women also need to reach emotional and cognitive (thinking) levels before they are ready to let go and relax into eroticism.

Getting a woman to this point can take time. Sometimes it can take days! If you want to have sex with a woman on a Saturday, then you might have to start on a Wednesday! You have learned in earlier chapters some ways to make this happen. Again, what that might look like could include the following:

- Coming up behind her as she stands by the sink and kissing her neck.
- Sending her small notes through e-mail or text messages, reminding her of how much you are looking forward to sex with her on Saturday.
- Describing in detail the things you want to do to her when you have your sex date.
- Whispering in her ear before she goes to sleep how much she turns you on.
- Bringing her a small gift, perhaps a rose, to tell her how you value her and your sexual relationship.
- Having a sex date. See exercise on page 178.

These things will help the woman look forward to the sex date. Anticipation is a great aphrodisiac.

EXERCISE
Sex Date

Make a date with your partner for sex. Four days prior to the date, use small acts to create anticipation for the big night. For example, show your partner physical affection at least three times the first day. Attempt to connect on the second day by whispering in your partner's ear the things you want to do to him or her on your sex date. On the third day, bring home a surprise. This can be something like a card or small token gift. The surprise might be something you can use on your sex date.

The fourth day is the big day, so create an atmosphere in the bedroom that will remind both of you that this is a sacred, erotic space for you to play safely in together. Light candles, put fresh flowers in the room and put soft sheets and blankets on the bed. Make an extra effort to pick out music that your partner will like.

When the big night comes, keep your expectations open and reasonable. If the evening goes well, then great. If it doesn't live up to your expectations, remember that this night can be anything that works for you and makes you feel connected to your partner. Massage, communication, and sharing fantasies using the Imago dialogue can make this an important night of sensual pleasures.

3. Emotional reminders. The need to be reminded about the connection with one's partner is not unique to women, but for women to feel relaxed and comfortable and to have a deepening of their erotic connection, they need to be reminded that they are safe. The way for male partners to do this is by reminding their women that they are still loved. Women say things to men like, "Do you still love me? Are you sure you love me?" which can sometimes be annoying for their partner.

As one man said in a sex workshop, "I told her I loved her when we got married. Isn't that enough for her? Why does she need to hear it again?"

Although this is an extreme example, it illustrates the point that men sometimes assume that their partner should know how they feel based on past conversations. But women need to be reminded, and often. It's not that they forget; it's that the reassurance of hearing it repeated on a regular basis helps them to relax into the security of the relationship. Testing the boundaries of their safety is part of what helps women to relax and surrender, knowing that their relationship has strong boundaries and will contain all of their fears and needs.

4. Permission. Because of women's guilt and shame around sex, there may be times when women don't feel that they deserve to have sexual pleasure. If there is sexual abuse in their pasts, or imagined fears that prevent letting go, then having "permission" to let go can help.

Some women don't feel like they deserve pleasure of any kind. This happens when they feel overly responsible in their lives. Their partners can tell them: "You deserve this break. You work so hard, you deserve to have all the pleasure I can give you."

5. Safety to surrender. When women receive permission, they often feel safer to surrender to the erotic moment. If they know that their partner is directive and in charge, they can relax into the experience, knowing someone is going to create an atmosphere that will help them feel like they can let go. This surrender is very important for orgasm.

There does not have to be total safety to have erotic sex or passion in a relationship. A slight bit of anxiety can heighten the anticipation and create more erotic drama for women. People are sometimes addicted to this level of excitement and arousal and look for ways to create it in their lives. The drama or crisis that is created sometimes adds an element of eroticism, particularly if there is danger or a sense of the forbidden involved.

But if the drama is risking the safety of the relationship, then it becomes toxic to a passionate partnership. This level of stimulation can be created within the partnership by planning sex that is risky or slightly scary. If women feel safe then they will not only feel turned on but will also be able to totally surrender.

6. The language of love. The way to know a woman's love language is to ask her! The languages of love are the same for women as they are for men. Finding out what her love language is can help her feel loved. Knowing her needs can help you fulfill her and give her what she wants. This is an act of generosity that shows you care about her.

The Language of Love for Women

In this exercise, we'll discover and explore how to love our partners in a way that makes them feel loved. You will need a pen and paper for this exercise.

Step One

Write down five things your partner did in the beginning of the relationship that made you feel loved. Write down five things he or she does now to make you feel loved. (There may be some overlap in these things, or they may be all new.)

Step Two

Take a look at your list and see what kind of love language you have. You may be closer to understanding your own language of love now. Which category does your love language fall under? Do you appreciate time, sex, praise, acts of service, or gifts?

Share the list with your partner. Ask for one thing that you would like your partner to do that makes you feel loved. Have your partner ask the same of you.

Step Three

Commit to fulfilling that language of love behavior at least once in the coming week.

Step Four

Meet again to talk about how it felt to get that need met. Make sure you tell your partner how much you appreciated him or her for doing this for you and making you feel loved.

Different Sexual Styles

David Schnarch, author of *Passionate Marriage,* says that there are three different types of sex—trance sex, partner engagement, and role-play.

People who are into trance sex need to shut off all outside stimulation to experience their pleasure and sensation. Being engaged with your partner means feeling emotional, intimate, and connected with your partner through sex. Role-play sex is about acting out and talking during sex. The following case illustrates how we can have different sexual styles and how at times these styles can feel confusing because they are different than our own needs. Learning more about how our partner operates sexually will help increase our understanding of what he or she needs in bed.

Dawn and Damien came into my office because of their difficulty pleasing each other during sex.

Damien: "When Dawn has sex, she doesn't want any outside stimulation. She wants to close her eyes, she doesn't want noise or talking, and sometimes she puts a pillow over her eyes or hides her face in her arm."

Dawn: "Well, I don't like it when Damien talks all the time. He is into this role-play thing and wants to talk during sex, and he wants me to talk to him."

Damien: "If she would just go along sometimes with what I want, I would love it. But she gets all embarrassed and the mood is shot. I just don't even want to try anymore."

I asked them what they had done in the past to work on their sex life.

Damien: "I bought Dawn an outfit, I have brought home porn movies, and I have tried to have sex with her in unusual places, like that time in the parking lot at my office."

Damien was a "role-play" type of sexual person. He wanted to talk during sex and was turned on when Dawn talked to him. He didn't need her to become something she wasn't, but he wanted a more active type of sex that included imagination, sex games, and playing roles during sex.

Dawn, on the other hand, was a "trance" type of sexual person. She needed to block out all outside stimulation so that she could totally focus on the sensations in her body. She was only able to orgasm if she could get lost in the experience and feel every nuance of their lovemaking.

The need for "partner engagement" includes a need to gaze into a partner's eyes during sex. When Damien asked Dawn to keep her eyes open, she would lose interest in the sex. She would pull away and they would both be angry and hurt. Neither of these preferences is wrong. However, not knowing the other's style in bed had created an atmosphere where neither had a fulfilling experience.

For couples to enjoy each other and create passion in their partnership they have to understand each other's style. At times each partner needs to push his or her edge (or limits) to try the other's style of sex. To maintain desire, both partners have to experience the other as someone who is willing and able to come to their side of the bed, and to act out their erotic fantasies. Being willing to try sex in other ways is what makes passion possible.

Use Sexual Anatomy Knowledge to Improve Your Sex Life

8

Most of the sex education handouts in our grade school health classes are of internal reproductive organs. That education is very necessary, but so is the more specific education about our sexual organs and their unique responses to stimulation and desire.

Sexual desire, and what to do about it, is not taught in school. Girls are not taught what to do when they feel an attraction to the boy sitting next to them in math class. Boys are not taught what to do with their intense sexual urges that peak in adolescence. Both boys and girls, as they reach adolescence, begin a stumbling around process that signifies the beginning of their experimentation with sex. The "backseat fumble," the reach under the T-shirt, the furtive kisses behind the ice cream shop: all of these experiences are the beginning of a journey toward erotic partnership.

To empower girls to make choices based on self-respect and integrity, they must be taught how to recognize their desires so that they can be expressed when the time feels right. Girls also need to learn about boys' sexuality. For boys to feel in control of their sexuality and to move into relationships without guilt and shame, they need education in mutual sexual desire.

Many of us are not taught about desire or what to do when we feel like acting out our feelings. Many women are confused about their body's sexual signals, which makes it hard for them to communicate their sexual needs. If women don't recognize their own erotic desires, they begin to split off from their sexuality, become dissociated during sex, and feel frustrated and dissatisfied. Men can be confused about when and how to act on their desires, and not understand a woman's sometimes confusing signals.

Test Your Knowledge

The following quiz will help you begin to identify what you know about your own sexual anatomy and that of your partner. As you take the quiz and answer the questions, notice what you are curious about. Then, after reading the rest of the chapter, take the quiz again and see how much you have learned!

Knowing about your sexual anatomy and how your body works can help you discover the endless wonders of your own sexuality. Learning about your partner's sexual anatomy and how his or her body works can help you have the sex you have always wanted.

In Imago therapy, we learn that our growth lies in what we bring *to* the relationship, not what we get *out* of it. When we give our partners what they really want, we grow into fully realized individuals.

EXERCISE
Sexual Anatomy Quiz

Answer the following questions together with your partner or separately and see how well you each score. Then, take the quiz again after reading this chapter and compare your scores. Remember, you will be testing yourselves to see how much you have learned from reading this chapter.

1. How long do women take to achieve orgasm after direct clitoral stimulation?

   3 to 5 minutes? 8 to 10 minutes? 7 to 20 minutes? 15 to 30 minutes?

2. Where is the perineum located on women?

3. Where is the perineum located on men?

4. Where is the G-spot on women located?

5. The G-spot is actually the root of what part of the body?

6. Where is the male prostate gland located?

7. The male prostate gland is similar in nerve structure to which part of the female anatomy?

8. What is more stimulating, labia massage or clitoral massage?

9. Out of what orifice does a woman urinate?

10. Can a man orgasm without ejaculating?

11. Can a woman ejaculate while having an orgasm?

12. Are there pleasure centers in the anus?

13. What are clitoral roots?

The Ways We Become Aroused

One of the first things we need to know about sexual anatomy is that there are similarities and differences in how men and women become sexually stimulated.

Men and women both get aroused by these types of stimulation:

- **Visual.** If we are stimulated visually, then we are aroused by what we see. We will be stimulated by what our partners look like. We will get turned on by watching them. It will stimulate us to watch them having sex. We may also get aroused by watching pornography or seeing erotic photos.

- **Touch or kinesthetic.** The feel of things on our bodies is arousing. If we are kinesthetic, then touch engages us sexually more than our other senses do. Touching our partners, feeling their skin, and being held will be important to us for experiencing pleasure. Massage, feathers, feather dusters, ice cubes, and any other stimulation that creates a kinesthetic response will make us feel passionate and alive.

- **Auditory.** If we are auditory, then the sounds of lovemaking will get us excited. Listening to the soft sounds of our partner's pleasure or hearing them scream with passion will send us over the edge. Sexy music, poetry read out loud, and hearing our partners "talk dirty" will turn us on.

- **Thought or cognitive.** The stimulation of our imagination can also be arousing. Having fantasies in our minds will get us hot. Thinking about our partners and imagining them in different positions or having erotic fantasies about them will stimulate the cognitive mind.

The difference between men and women is primarily seen in their responses to arousal. Men have one level of arousal, and usually want to be touched immediately and can get an erection with little prompting. Men can go from feeling aroused to orgasm in a relatively short time. They peak, and they begin to come down almost immediately, which is why men often fall asleep after their orgasm.

For women, plateaus of arousal take longer, and there are more of them. While arousal may take a while, women can stay at higher levels of arousal for longer periods of time, allowing for multiple orgasms and a more gradual descent back to normal. This is why women need foreplay and why they stay in a sexually aroused place for a long period of time after an orgasm.

We will talk later about ways for men to stay in the higher plateaus of arousal, going from plateau to plateau and staying erect without reaching orgasm.

What We Do When We're Aroused

You may feel physical responses when you feel desire, but you do not have to act on any of them. You have a choice about what to do with your desires. When you feel sexually aroused, you have several options:

- You can act out with another person
- You can self-stimulate
- You can fantasize
- You can sublimate
- You can avoid your feelings

Acting out with another person means engaging in sex. Self-stimulation refers to masturbation and self-pleasure. Fantasizing is anything in your mind that brings erotic imagery. To sublimate your arousal means to work it out through some other positive behavior, like creating artwork or playing music.

Avoiding your feelings is perhaps the most risky option, since it implies that your feelings *can* be avoided. Feelings need to be expressed and can come out at a later time when we least expect it.

EXERCISE
Learning about Stimulation

For this exercise, find some quiet time to answer the following questions. Both men and women should take this quiz, as it applies to both sexes. You will need some time afterward to process your answers with your partner in an Imago dialogue, using mirroring, validation, and empathy.

Answer "true" or "false" to each of the following questions and share your answers with your partner:

- If I felt more comfortable in my body I think I would have sex more often.
- I recognize when my body is responding to stimulation, either visual, physical, or in my thoughts.
- I am a visually stimulated person.
- I am primarily stimulated by physical touch.
- I use my imagination to stimulate myself sexually.
- I often feel my body's signals for sexual desire.
- I would like to feel my body's signals for sexual desire.
- I like the feel of garments and materials around me, such as scarves, sweaters, etc.
- I like to have nice sheets and blankets on my bed.
- I love to take bubble baths and wear perfumes and scented creams on my body.
- I get manicures and pedicures often.
- I let people massage me and enjoy healthy nonsexual touch.

Looking at your answers, what did you notice about yourself? Share your answers with your partner, reading out loud the question and whether you answered "true" or "false." Have your partner mirror back what you say. Then your partner will validate by responding, "It makes sense you would like X because I know you like to feel X." Then your partner empathizes by guessing at one feeling he or she thinks this gives you. For example, "I imagine you feel very relaxed and sexy when you take a hot bubble bath." Then share anything you learned about your partner after hearing his or her answers.

The Avenue to Anal Stimulation

The anus has similar responses to the vagina during sex. It contracts during an orgasm in the same way the vagina does. There are lots of nerve endings in the anus, so that receiving anal stimulation can feel great if done with lots of lubricant and communication with your partner.

Be aware that receiving anal stimulation can be both pleasurable and painful. The internal and external sphincter muscles tighten and relax, controlling the passage to the anus. These muscles must be relaxed for something to enter externally.

To create the possibility of anal sex, your partner needs to work with you to help you relax. Exploring this sensitive area can include a combination of massage, lubrication, and relaxation techniques including deep breathing. Sex toys that are narrower than a finger can be used at first to test the anus's response to insertion. Make sure the anal toy is wider at the base, to prevent it from going too far into the rectum. The anus will suck things into it when it tightens, and these things may not come out. Be careful that anything you insert into the anus and rectum will be easy to retrieve.

Using good communication, couples can talk to each other during this experience to explore what feels good and what is uncomfortable. Stopping immediately when the discomfort gets too dramatic is an important thing to agree on prior to any anal play. Knowing your partner is sensitive to your body and what feels good will increase the trust between you.

Getting to Know
Our Bodies

Having an orgasm for women is sometimes complicated. When they are out of touch with their bodies, women can have a hard time figuring out what gives them pleasure.

Some women at midlife have never had an orgasm, although many have faked one. And faking orgasm is confusing to men, since they don't know which signals to trust or how to create sensations for women that will lead to a real orgasm!

Even as adults, women can be ignorant of how their bodies work. Lots of women think they urinate from their vaginas. Most women have never looked at their genitals in a mirror.

Without embarrassment, can you tell your partner, with the most direct and graphic language possible, the location of your different body parts? Can you give him or her an anatomy lesson? Perhaps you will tell your partner things he or she already knows, or you may explain your body in a way that makes it a new discovery for your partner.

Try to explain to your partner what you need to achieve an orgasm and then ask your partner what kind of stimulation he or she needs to have an orgasm. Share what feels good to each of you.

This next exercise should help you teach your partner about your body and what gives you pleasure.

EXERCISE
Playing Doctor

As a passionate partner, learning about sexual anatomy, (what is where and how to use it), is an important part of being a fully present and empathetic lover. Understanding each other's anatomy leads to new journeys of exploration and connection.

For this exercise, you will need at least sixty minutes of uninterrupted time together. Make sure the room is warm and comfortable. Put on soft music and low lights, but with enough illumination to really see and appreciate your partner's body.

(continued on page 190)

(continued)

Remember, as you verbalize this information with your partner, you will use the Imago dialogue method of mirroring, so that everything your partner shares with you becomes an opportunity to help him or her feel heard and seen.

Step One

Choose who will be the sender and who will be the receiver. Senders should ask their partners (receivers) to show them all the parts of their body. Receivers should explain how these parts work and what they feel like. Senders mirror back what their partners say. Ask questions as if you were seeing these parts for the first time. Mirror back the answers.

Step Two

Senders should ask their partners what happens in specific places in their body during arousal and orgasm. Senders mirror back what they hear. Ask them how their body parts feel when they are aroused, which parts of their anatomy feel the best when caressed, and how they like to be touched in those places. Senders should mirror what they hear.

Step Three

Switch, and senders now explain to the receivers all their parts, showing and pointing to the more hidden locations so that their partners can see clearly what is happening in the sender's body.

Senders should tell receivers what stimulation their body parts need to become aroused. Receivers should mirror what they hear. Senders should explain what type of touch feels the best on what part, what happens as they get closer to orgasm, and where they feel their orgasm. Receivers should mirror what they hear.

Step Four

Thank your partner for sharing this very intimate experience with you! Share with each other what you appreciated about this exercise, mirroring back what you hear. Move into sexual play, pleasure, or intercourse if that feels right for you both in this moment. Otherwise, enjoy the appreciations and new knowledge of each other's body!

Anatomy 101: Female Genitalia

For most of us, women's genitals are a mystery—even for women! The majority of women never look at their genitals with a mirror. And since most women don't normally see other women's genitals, their own anatomy can remain a mystery.

We see men's genitals all the time. They are on statues and in fine art everywhere. Like the female breast, the penis has been immortalized in stone and in paint for centuries. But the female equivalent, the vulva, is not a popular subject of artwork. Just by virtue of the fact that the female genitalia remain hidden anatomically, women don't get a chance to see what other vulvas look like. We don't see women's vulvas in the locker room. Not all vaginas are alike. They differ as widely as penis shapes do.

Here's a rundown of what you should know about female genitalia, including the famed G-spot.

The **vulva** consists of two sets of **labia**, or lips. The word *labia* is derived from the Latin word meaning "lips." The outer lips, *labia majora*, are what we see if a woman is shaved or has no hair on her vulva. The inner lips, the inner labia or *labia minora*, are smaller and thinner, protect the opening of the vagina, and are extremely sensitive. Labia or lips are folds of skin that vary in size and elasticity. Not all labia look alike! They are as unique to the individual as any other part of a woman's body. The labia swell when aroused. Sometimes the inner labia hang outside the outer labia and sometimes they are covered. Both are normal.

Looking at a woman directly while she is lying on her back, the vulva is slightly pear-shaped, with the narrower part on top and the wider parts at the bottom. Or it can be narrow at both ends and wider in the middle. Inside the inner labia the **clitoris** (klit-er-iss) is at the top. The opening to the vagina is in the wider part of the vulva. In between the clitoris and the vagina is the **urethra**. The urethra is the opening where women urinate. Women do not urinate from their vagina, even during orgasm.

The **clitoris** is a small projection, approximately the size of a pea, situated above the vagina, at the top of the vulva. The clitoris can project out from between the labia minora or be hidden in the folds of the labia. Women's clitoral size varies. It can be anywhere from the size of the tip of a pinky finger to two inches long.

The **anus** is below the vagina, and the **perineum** is the area in between the bottom of the vagina and the anus.

When touching a vulva, always have clean hands. Go slowly at first, and be gentle. Touching the sensitive parts of the vulva using dry fingers can catch and drag the skin and feel uncomfortable, so use a water-based lubricant.

The urethra is sensitive to bacteria, and nothing should be dragged or rubbed over this area that might have bacteria from the anus or dirt from fingers or hands. Lubricants with scents or heating effects can cause urinary tract or yeast infections. Any chemical that comes into contact with this area can cause burning, discomfort, and infection.

The **frenulum** of the clitoris is the skin that attaches it to the body. Like a penis, the clitoris becomes erect when it is aroused. There is a "hood" or **prepuce** over the clitoris, which is skin that covers and hugs the clitoris and pulls back as the clitoris becomes erect. When erect, the clitoris is very sensitive and cannot normally be rubbed directly.

Like the penis for men, the clitoris is the center of sexual arousal for women. It has the highest concentration of nerve endings in the body, and is the seat of pleasure on a woman's body. Stimulating the clitoris is the secret to pleasing a woman and giving her an orgasm.

The clitoris extends upward and to the back, before splitting into two parts called the **crura**, or clitoral *roots*. It can extend its shaft up inside the body and can be as long as five inches internally. The roots extend around and into the interior of the labia. These two bundles of nerves and tissue can extend deep into the vaginal walls, or they can be connected closer to the surface of the labia. It is possible that the clitoris has its primary root or origin in the G-spot, which is anatomically behind the clitoris and located in the vagina.

The clitoral roots actually extend internally all the way down and around both sides of the vagina, into the perineum, and down to the anus. These roots can be stimulated and enhance sensations leading to orgasm.

The inner and outer sections of the clitoris, and its extensions or roots down around the vagina, make the clitoris similar in structure to the penis, with the clitoris mirroring the sensitive head of the male penis.

The G-Spot

Famed German gynecologist Ernst Grafenberg "found" the **G-spot** in 1950, and it was aptly named after him for his discovery. Grafenberg described this area as a possible "second internal clitoris." Many refuted the idea, questioning the existence of the G-spot at all. Others have claimed that it is the "back side" of the clitoris, while current research is trying to prove that the G-spot is probably home to the ultimate roots of the clitoris.

The G-spot is an area two inches inside the front wall of the vagina, behind the pubic bone. When stimulated through the vagina, the G-spot expands or swells upon arousal. The G-spot has a different texture than the rest of the vagina. It can feel smoother or rougher than the vaginal walls. It can also feel like a spongy area, and be anywhere from the size of a pea to the size of a half-dollar coin. The G-spot can be stimulated to create heightened levels of arousal and, for many women, vaginal orgasm.

One way to know that you have found the G-spot is when pressure on the area creates a pressure to urinate. The G-spot is located just above the bladder and can press on the urethra. If this feeling can be tolerated, the area will continue to respond and more intense pressure can be applied.

Stimulating the G-Spot

G-spot orgasm can be intense and actually trigger strong emotional responses, like crying. Doing G-spot massage and concentrating on this area should be done with respect and sensitivity, so that any and all feelings can become part of the experience.

The good news about G-spot orgasms is that women can have one before, during, or after a clitoral orgasm. Before women recover from a clitoral orgasm, stimulation to her G-spot can trigger another orgasm.

The good news about
G-spot orgasms is that women can have one before, during, or after a clitoral orgasm.

The stimulation can feel intense when a woman is already engorged and throbbing from the clitoral response. Women can have multiple orgasms in this way, or go up close to the point of orgasm and come back down again, riding the wave to the ultimate climax. This experience not only triggers strong emotions but can also induce an almost trancelike state, similar to meditation but more blissful.

G-spot orgasms can be explosive. Some women emit a vaginal fluid that can actually squirt out of the vagina at the time of orgasm. Some women will experience this female ejaculation during a G-spot orgasm. Female ejaculate is a clear fluid and is not urine. It is not created in the bladder, but emanates from the vaginal walls themselves.

A G-spot orgasm can take longer than a clitoral orgasm. Vaginal climax only happens when the clitoris is aroused simultaneously, either directly or indirectly. This can happen when the clitoris is stimulated by direct touching, by rubbing the clitoral roots in the labia and opening to the vagina, or by stimulating the clitoris through the G-spot.

The G-spot is engorged when it is aroused. It can't be found unless the woman is already turned on. Trying to rub or caress the G-spot before a woman is totally stimulated can sometimes cause discomfort or pain.

Vaginal and clitoral orgasms feel different. During a vaginal orgasm, there is a pushing down sensation in the vagina and cervix, and the contractions push out. Women might even push out their lover's penis or fingers! When women have a clitoral orgasm, there is a suction effect created by the contractions, and the pulsing of the muscles will squeeze from inside.

The partner stimulating the G-spot needs to know that this is a wonderful experience and should be honored. However, a vaginal orgasm is not always possible. Partners will need to use more pressure and time to stimulate the vagina or G-spot to orgasm, compared to the stimulation needed for a clitoral orgasm. For most women, stimulating the vagina alone is like stimulating only the scrotum on a man. It feels nice, but is not likely to get them off.

How to Stimulate the Clitoris

Because the clitoris is so sensitive, it must be approached with tenderness and sensitivity. Some women can tolerate stronger and deeper pressure as they become more aroused. A good rule of thumb for partners is to start by applying well-lubricated pressure in a circular motion around the clitoris.

When the clitoris is aroused it will become engorged, erect, and more visible. Just prior to orgasm it actually rises up so that it may look like it is disappearing back into the folds of skin above and around it. This is an indication that orgasm is approaching.

Using the clock exercise in chapter 7, partners should try sliding their fingers around the clitoris in a circle, starting at twelve o'clock. Determine where the clitoris is the most responsive.

Experiment with gentle light flicking or pulling, kissing or soft biting, squeezing and pinching as the clitoris becomes more and more stimulated. Working with your partner, communicate exactly what is happening in your body, and tell your partner what you are feeling.

Use this next exercise to teach both partners where your clitoris is most sensitive and responsive to stimulation.

EXERCISE
Clitoris Play

For this exercise (an extension of "Clitoral Clock"), you'll need a warm room, and a bed, couch, or pillows on which to lie. Women should lie back, open their legs to their partner to receive soft stimulation, and keep their eyes open to gaze at their lover. The sender should apply water-based lubrication to his or her fingers.

For the partner stimulating the clitoris, start with gentle strokes on the inside of the thighs. Move closer to the vulva, lightly stroking the outer labia. Using deeper strokes, begin massaging the labia, sliding your well-lubricated fingers over the

(continued on page 196)

(continued)

inner and outer labia and getting into the outer area or threshold of the vagina. This will stimulate the area and you may feel the labia swelling or becoming engorged. The vagina may become naturally wet and lubricated, or a finger can be used to smooth lubricant into the outer opening of the vagina.

Begin pinching the labia between the palms of your hands, using longer strokes to stretch toward and gently stroke the clitoris. Come back to the vagina and down to the anal area, stimulating the perineum and the whole vulva area. Move up again to the clitoris, creating a teasing and a buildup of sensation. Insert a finger into the vagina occasionally, using a "come hither" motion to swipe the G-spot area, and come back to the clitoris. Wind around the clitoris with your finger using the clock motion. Ask your partner to make a noise or use words to describe when you are hitting supersensitive spots that feel great.

For many women, touching the top-left quadrant of the clitoris feels great. Try it, moving your fingers in tighter and tighter circles around the clitoris, leaning your palm on the vaginal area or using your other hand to stimulate the G-spot area inside the vagina.

Continue the clitoral stimulation for at least ten to fifteen minutes. Try a windshield wiper movement with two fingers over the clitoris, waving them back and forth, as your other hand is inserting a finger into the vagina and stimulating the G-spot.

Know that each of you can move around and adjust if you are getting cramps or feel uncomfortable. But keep coming back to the clitoral area, watching for signs that she is ready to orgasm.

Ask her now to tell you exactly what to do to bring her to orgasm. Have her use words or put her hand on yours to show you the exact move that will bring her over the edge. As she is coming, keep up the stimulation, although move softly on or around the clitoris. Stimulation at this point will feel very intense and can be uncomfortable.

Stopping too soon and discontinuing can also feel disconcerting. Some women like pressure or a finger inside their vagina as they come down from their orgasmic plateau.

Orgasm

The word orgasm is from the Greek word "orga," which means explosion. This makes sense because orgasm can feel like an explosion of pleasure and bliss. It is not uncommon for women to cry during or after orgasm, as the experience liberates stress and withheld emotions.

Women can orgasm for as long as twenty seconds. The intensity of the orgasm can vary, depending on G-spot, vaginal or clitoral stimulation.

Interestingly, a study from the Netherlands found that the area of the brain that controlled fear and anxiety was switched off during orgasm. This may indicate that letting go and surrendering is the easiest way to bring yourself to orgasm. The result is that feelings of fear and anxiety decrease.

Each woman will have her own wealth of knowledge regarding her body and what she needs to orgasm. No matter what the studies say, each woman is her own orgasm expert, the one who knows best what kind of stimulation and situations lead her to climax.

Anatomy 101: Male Genitalia

The **penis** is a highly sensitive area, with several parts—the **shaft**, the **glans** (or **head**), and the **scrotum**.

The glans of the penis is the most sensitive area, with the ridge surrounding the helmet shape being the most sensitive. The urethra is the opening at the head of the penis, and men can urinate when soft or erect. Men do not urinate and ejaculate at the same time.

The shaft is rigid during erection and soft when not erect. An uncircumcised penis has skin that reaches up and over the head of the penis. When the penis is erect, the foreskin, or skin covering the head, pulls back and the head is exposed.

The foreskin is removed at the time of circumcision. Both circumcised and uncircumcised penises are stimulated in the same way.

The scrotum is a soft, sensitive sack that holds the testicles. The scrotum has many nerve endings that can feel very pleasurable when stimulated. The testicles are kept warm and fertile in this sack, allowing an environment for sperm to thrive.

Men become erect during stimulation, and also involuntarily at times during REM sleep. Most stimulation feels good on a man's penis, and yet communicating about what feels the best can lead to a more positive experience for couples.

Try the following exercise as a way of finding out what kind of stimulation works best on your partner's penis.

EXERCISE
The Penis as a Work of Art

Take at least forty-five minutes for this exercise. Find a quiet, comfortable place where you will not be interrupted. For this exercise you will need markers (water-based) or different colored foods.

Men should take washable, water-based markers—scented ones are fine, too—and choose colors that represent sensation. You'll use these colors on your penis to show your partner which areas are the most sensitive to touch. For example, red can indicate the most sensitive area, green can show areas that feel good when touched, and yellow might show areas where you are the least sensitive.

Stimulate your penis to erection, using masturbation or your partner's manual manipulation. Using lubricant or saliva at this point will make it difficult to see the markers and decrease their efficacy. You will color small areas, about half an inch, directly on your penis.

Use different colors to show your partner the areas that feel the most sensitive and where you want to be touched. Do this exercise with your partner, drawing on these areas while your partner watches, or have your partner draw with the markers where you indicate.

Notice the beautiful work of art you both have created as your penis becomes a canvas of pleasure. If you have scented or flavored markers, your partner can lick off the colors, starting with the least sensitive areas and moving to the red hot zones. You can use food for this exercise as well, such as chocolate or strawberry sauce, whipped cream, or jelly.

Note: Make sure you wash off the marker before penetration to prevent possible infection.

The Prostate and Ancestors of Anal Beads

The prostate is a gland located internally in men. The prostate gland or "P-spot" is above the perineum and inside the anal wall. This area has as many nerve endings as the woman's G-spot and is many times equivalent in sensitivity.

The prostate secretes fluid into semen prior to ejaculation and controls the mobility of sperm. This fluid helps the sperm swim up the vagina and into the cervix, and keeps them viable long enough to connect with the egg in a woman's uterus. As men age or if there is prostate dysfunction, this fluid can decrease, and ejaculate amounts will also decrease. This does not influence the amount of sperm, but it can reduce their life span.

The prostate, when stimulated, enhances pleasure for men and can cause orgasm and ejaculation. Seventeenth-century sailors discovered this secret from the courtesans and prostitutes on the Orient shores where they landed. Sailors would request the ships that made runs to the Orient, because they knew that these women could stimulate them to ejaculation quickly and get them back on the ships before they left port.

These women developed a technique where they tied knots in silk scarves and inserted the scarf into a sailor's anus, then pulled it out slowly, stimulating their prostate. During orgasm, the knots would pull past their prostate and out of their anal sphincter muscles, creating intense waves of orgasmic pleasure. These scarves are the ancestors of plastic anal beads available today in sex toy stores and catalogs. The toys serve the same purpose, to stimulate the prostate as well as the anus itself.

The prostate has as many
nerve endings as the woman's G-spot
and is many times equivalent in sensitivity.

There are two ways to stimulate the prostate. One is to insert a well-lubricated finger into the anus and reach up about two inches, feeling for a round ball approximately the size of a golf ball. The prostate can be smaller or larger, depending on health and heredity.

Before inserting a finger into the anus, make sure you have lots of water-based lubricant on your finger and around the anal area. Go slowly, and only with permission.

Some men are hesitant about letting themselves feel the powerful sensations of prostate pleasure if they equate anal pleasure with homosexuality. Some men have shame and embarrassment about anal stimulation, although most men, if it is done correctly, will enjoy the sensations.

The second way to stimulate the prostate is through prostate massage. Because the prostate sits on the perineum, the area between the scrotum and the anus, outer massage can be done without going through the anus. Using lubricant, so the skin will not become irritated, massage with firm pressure. You may feel the shape of the prostate and you can massage to the depth that feels comfortable. With the right stimulation, this can be a very pleasurable experience for a man. Try this next exercise to stimulate the prostate.

EXERCISE
Prostate Massage

For this exercise you need at least sixty minutes of uninterrupted, safe time together. Make sure you will not have distractions or worries about children or responsibilities at this time.

Create a setting that reflects the mood you would like to have for this exercise. Soft rock, jazz, or classical music can be played in the background. Lower the lights, but not enough so you can't see one another.

Step One

Have the male partner lie on his back, knees bent. Ask him whether you may put your finger in the opening of his anus. Insert a well-lubricated finger into his anus and slide your finger slowly inside, feeling for the round shape of the prostate about two inches inside. Move your fingers in a "come hither" motion along the wall of the rectum that faces the front of his body.

Step Two

Stimulate his penis by rubbing it with your other hand, which should also be well lubricated, up and down, paying special attention to the head. As you slowly maneuver your finger deeper into his anus, if so, continue the "come hither" motion. Use your finger to gently massage the prostate.

Step Three

Ask him whether these motions feel good. Try several different strokes and pressures, asking him which feels better. Try squeezing his scrotum gently. Give him choices, such as "does this feel better, or this?"

Step Four

Put his penis in your mouth and keep massaging his prostate with your finger. Ask him to tell you when he is ready to come. Have him take a deep breath when you feel he is getting ready. If his penis is making jerking motions up toward his body or if he swells to a hard erection, he is getting ready to climax. Tell him to bear down on your finger, pushing your finger out of his anus. The combination of sensations will drive him crazy with pleasure.

Sexual Massage for Him and Her

All kinds of massage can be used to relax and awaken erotic feelings. The beginning of reexperiencing positive and generous touching can start with back rubs and body massage and move to massage of specific sexual parts.

These next three exercises will show you how to massage, stimulate, and pleasure your partner. These are direct contact exercises, where you will need lots of privacy and water-based lubricant. Make sure the room is warm and lit with candles or other soft light. You want adequate time to focus on pleasing your partner and uninterrupted space to feel relaxed and fully present for these erotic encounters.

EXERCISE
For Her: Labia Massage

Using lots of water-based lubricant, explore your partner's labia, both the inner and outer lips, using different techniques and strokes.

Put your palms together and slide the vulva between your hands. Smooth the vulva down and then back up with the palm of your hand. Using your fingertips, gently push into the area, massaging each side separately. Massage with your fingers slowly from the crease in the leg to the vagina, and go back out again. Combine labia massage strokes with strokes over and around the clitoris, vagina, and anus. Be careful to keep any fingers that touch the anus away from the rest of the vulva.

Massage the clitoris and vaginal area to orgasm, or just use this massage experience as a way to give and receive pleasure and sensation. Massage can be a wonderful way to connect with your partner, and it does not need to lead to the "finish line." Sometimes pleasuring each other can be the goal.

EXERCISE
For Him: Scrotum Licking

For men, scrotum licking can be an intense experience that brings joy and pleasure.

Using your tongue, bathe the scrotum in saliva, tasting each area of the scrotum from the inner leg to the perineum and back to the base of the penis. Play with the sack and testicles inside of it gently. Take one testicle in your mouth at a time and suck it gently, lubricating it with your saliva and your tongue. Lick all around the scrotum and then slide to the penis with your mouth.

Now using lubricant, massage the whole area from the base of the penis to the perineum. Make sure that you use a firm grip, at times gently pulling or rolling the scrotum sack. Never yank or pull too hard.

EXERCISE
For Both: Perineum Massage

The perineum is the area from the vagina to the anus on women and the area from the scrotum to the anus on men. These areas can be massaged and bring prostate stimulation to men and possibly some clitoral stimulation for women.

Start with lots of lubricant and experiment with different pressures, from a light scratch or tickle with your fingertips to harder movements and strokes. Try rubbing and pressing with your palm, and ask your partner what he or she would like more of.

This can be a wonderful way to connect your partner to his or her root, the base of the perineum, where there is a lot of power and energy. That energy can be drawn up into the genitals, the belly, and the heart. In the next chapter we will talk more about sex and spirituality and how to combine the anatomical moves with breathing and meditation.

Women's Struggle with Body Image

For women, sex with a passionate partner can be the beginning of waking up and reexperiencing being totally present in the body. As women become more open about their need for sex, they may be faced with feelings about their own bodies.

Most women today are concerned with their appearance and worry about how they look naked. Only 5 percent of women fit the standard ideal for models in this country—the average woman is 140 pounds, 5'4", and a size 14. The modeling industry is made up of women whose average height is 5'10" and an average weight of 107 pounds. Feeling the pressure of our culture, our media, and the fashion industry, women find it difficult accepting and loving the body they are in.

There are new standards in the fashion industry, particularly in Spain and other parts of Europe, where models are required to have a healthy percentage of body fat on their frames before they can become fashion models. As these standards trigger change all over the world, women may feel less pressure to conform to an unrealistic standard.

The pressure to stay youthful in our society also makes women feel anxious to be in top physical shape and to fight aging through liposuction, Botox injections, and plastic surgery.

Most women polled say that if they felt more comfortable in their bodies they would have sex more often. Women can learn from this, by pushing their edge and trying to have sex even when they feel uncomfortable about their physical selves. (Notice how you feel after a wonderful lovemaking session. Are you less insecure about your body parts?)

Working on body image is an important part of a relationship, because being physically confident helps you bring your whole self to the relationship. Performing the following exercise when you have negative thoughts about your self-image can help you feel more accepting of your body.

EXERCISE
Accepting Your Body

Look in the mirror and repeat this affirmation ten times a day for two weeks: "I love and accept myself exactly as I am." You may notice that when you have a negative body thought, this phrase begins to come up instead. And over time you may actually come to believe it.

Every time a negative thought or self-doubt comes up, repeat the affirmation until it drives out the negative thought from your mind. Every time you have a less than complimentary thought about your looks, repeat the affirmation to yourself. This exercise will help replace negative thoughts with self-acceptance.

It is only through acceptance that you will learn to love your body. Good sex means being totally present and open without the need to hide any part of yourself.

Men's Struggle with Body Image

The need for sex is normal and natural for women and is important for body image recovery as well as healthy eating patterns. Many men have body image issues as well.

While women worry that they are not small enough, sometimes men feel insecure about not being big enough. Men feel pressure to appear muscular, particularly as they get older. As they lose their hair or gain weight around their waists, men can have a negative body image as well.

Men worry about how their bodies compare to those of other men. They have fears about whether or not they can satisfy their female partners. Mostly, they worry about their penis size. When men are asked what they would most like to change about their bodies, they say "hair, stomach, and a larger penis."

For men, having sex makes them more comfortable in their bodies. When men feel that their partner loves and appreciates their penis, it helps them to relax in their sexuality. Comparing their penis size to actors in porn movies makes men feel insecure. Male genitals in pornography are many times larger than the average-sized penis. Men can feel competitive over the size of their penis, and they need to know that their size and shape are perfect for you.

Letting your partner know the things you really like about his body can help. Praise him for the way he moves in his skin, for the way he uses his hands, for how good his hard chest feels against your soft body. Use your auditory skills to tell him how much you love his penis.

A way for both men and women to become more comfortable and appreciate their bodies in all their wonders is to learn how the body responds in its skin. Discovering what feels good sensually helps you value your body and feel connected to its sensual desires. The following exercise will help you begin to appreciate that your body is not just a clothing size or a number on the scale, but is a receptor for sensual delights.

EXERCISE
Getting in Touch with the Sensual World

Create sensuality for your body and your senses by trying some of these exercises:

- Wear soft clothes that feel sensual against your skin.
- Use soft sheets with a higher thread count and blankets that have a sensual touch, as well as soft pillows and comforters on your bed.
- Place soft throw pillows and blankets around you in your home.
- Light scented candles and add fresh flowers to your bedroom.
- Take a hot soapy bath with fragrant bath soaps and salts.
- Start massaging you body with scented lotions and creams.
- Add a manicure and pedicure to your weekly routine (men can get manicures and pedicures with a nail buff instead of polish).
- Brush your hair 100 times, just to feel the sensation on your scalp.
- Get a massage using scented and slippery massage oils.
- Try appreciating all of your physical sensual self.

A Lifetime of Passion

When you "wake up" a relationship and allow each partner to be present to the gifts of each other's fantasy life, you create a stronger, more committed partnership. To have this long-term passion, there needs to be healthy communication about sexual needs, including a way to deal with anger and resentment, such as channeling it into the sexual relationship.

Anger can be dysfunctional when it interferes with healthy sexuality. But it can also be channeled into a passionate sex life.

If there is anger in a relationship, there is energy. It means that the relationship is alive and awake. In a partnership, being "awake" includes a mutual sexual appreciation of each other, where you both feel seen and desired. When signs of "drowsiness" appear, the sexual energy in a relationship can be awakened using Imago therapy techniques.

In our society we like to say, "Never go to bed angry." The problem is that if we can't bring our anger into the bedroom in a constructive way, we put off a chance for two loving partners to resolve conflict.

Channeling resentment into your sexual relationship can be scary, but it solves several dilemmas. One, it allows relief from the stress of the conflict and it helps us trust that our partners are being honest about their feelings. If we can be connected to our partners even when they are angry, then there is less fear that anger will cause a permanent disconnection. If we withdraw from our partners when we are angry, we never resolve the problem, and we grow farther and farther apart.

Knowing that anger is okay takes some of the pressure off of the partnership. It is unrealistic to think that you will never be angry at your partner. Understanding what to do about anger and how to work through it is a way to build a permanent connection.

Being honest about your anger and expressing it in healthy, nonviolent ways can help you connect with your partner. (Note: Anger is healthy but violence is not. Make sure you get help if you are experiencing a violent relationship, either as the one inflicting violence or the one receiving it.)

Chemical Romance

When we are angry, we get a surge of the brain chemical adrenalin, which signals conflict to our bodies. But we don't have to wait until we work through our conflict to engage in sex. Other brain chemicals like oxytocin, dopamine, and serotonin are all released when we have sex, which makes us feel calmer and more attached to our partner.

When we first meet, we are attracted to a potential partner because of the serotonin levels that are triggered in our system. We feel a rush of good feelings and some obsessiveness, too. That is why we think about our new love all of the time. Longer-term attraction is created by higher levels of oxytocin, the feel-good chemical that is released after sex.

If the initial physical "serotonin attraction" wears off, it would seem you need more oxytocin in the relationship, which leads to long-term satisfaction. And because oxytocin is released in the body during and after sex, wouldn't it make sense that the more sex you have the more attracted to your partner you are for longer periods of time?

The more sex you have, the more of these "love hormones" you release. When you stop having sex, your body naturally lowers its estrogen and testosterone levels. So, having sex makes you want more sex. Sex is the ultimate aphrodisiac.

Maximizing versus Minimizing Anger

Without safety in a relationship there can be no true intimacy, either physical or emotional. Yet, stuffing your anger does not help your partner feel safe. Anger has a way of coming out sideways when we don't express it directly.

Passive-aggressive anger is resentment that is not direct, but is acted out in more subtle ways, such as coming home late, ignoring our partner, or withholding sex as a punishment. Withholding sex as a way to express resentment can be toxic to a good partnership.

This doesn't mean we shouldn't get angry—anger is a normal and natural response to frustration. What we do with our anger is the important issue. Most of us have conflict in our relationship at some time. When there is conflict, we react by **maximizing** or **minimizing** it. "Maximizers" have a tendency to create drama when they don't feel heard. This is their way of testing the bond of the partnership. They blow things out of proportion and dramatize their feelings. This can be a sign that what the maximizer is really craving is safety, not an argument! Maximizers test the walls of the box to make sure they are strong.

"Minimizers," on the other hand, are people who avoid conflict. They would rather withdraw from the problem and spend time alone to figure out an answer. They retreat into their emotional cave, fleeing the conflict or danger.

When a maximizer's partner retreats, the maximizer feels abandoned and pursues the minimizer, forcing this person deeper and farther into the cave. The more the maximizer pursues the minimizer, the more the minimizer persists in his or her pattern of responding—the fight escalates and both partners feel misunderstood.

Changing this pattern of defensive responses in your relationship can go a long way toward resolving conflict. For example, the best thing to do for minimizers is to give them space. For maximizers, this might be very difficult. If they can give minimizing partners a little time to process the conflict, they will come out on their own when they feel safe.

A minimizer can help a maximizer feel safe by staying present for the conflict for a little while longer than feels comfortable. Minimizers might want to retreat and hide out until the conflict passes, but if they can try something different and stay present for just a few extra moments, they can begin to change the pattern.

Responding to a Maximizer and a Minimizer

Learning how to have a "dialogue" instead of a conversation can go a long way toward helping maximizers feel safe. A dialogue helps maximizers feel that they are being heard. The maximizer feels dismissed when the minimizer says things like, "Why are we fighting over this? It's no big deal." A maximizer will react by saying things like, "You don't care how I feel."

How we respond is important. Instead of retreating during an argument, let the maximizer know, "Look, I am here, everything is good, you are safe. I can handle this. I am not going anywhere." This reassuring language can make a potential flare-up fizzle out.

When minimizers are angry they may withdraw, becoming uncommunicative and silently resentful. They don't want to be pursued and usually don't want to talk about the conflict. Minimizers aren't sure how to express their anger in healthy ways and many times would rather avoid it altogether. As stated above, giving minimizers space and time can help them gather their thoughts. And then it is important to let them know that anger can be talked about and that it is safe to come out of the cave!

We all act as minimizers and maximizers, depending on the issue, and this happens in all relationships. How we recognize this and respond to it is more important than trying to stop it. Try the next exercise as a way to step out of old fighting patterns.

EXERCISE
Containing Your Reactivity

Consider how you react when you are angry at your partner. What do you want to do? Walk away? Fight? Hide?

Whatever your reactivity is, your behavior when you are upset or angry at your partner is the behavior that scares him or her the most. It's hard to keep our reactive behavior in check. When we are scared or hurt we go into reactive, defensive behavior. Many times this looks like anger.

If you are a maximizer, you may find it challenging to hold back your reactivity, especially when you are angry. Minimizers may find it difficult to stay fully present when they feel anger.

Decide where your growth edge lies. Your growth edge is the area where you need to change your behavior. Knowing how you need to change and actually making those changes is how you grow. If you are unsure where your growth edge is, check with your partner. He or she usually knows where your growth lies.

Challenging your personal growth edge means pushing yourself into a new behavior, a new way of reacting when your partner gets angry. This may feel uncomfortable at first, especially in the middle of feeling the anger.

For this exercise, you will need to practice it when you are in a conflict. Next time you feel your reactive behavior kick in during a conflict, use a container exercise. This means pushing your edge of comfort, and staying uncomfortable for a few more moments than is normal for you. For instance, if your reactive behavior is to walk away during a conflict, engage your partner, talk, touch, and contain your feelings for one or more moments longer than you feel comfortable. Then walk away if you have to.

Do the same thing if you typically argue when you are angry—breathe, hold the feeling, talk, touch, and contain.

Each time you do this exercise you will be growing out of your usual behavior pattern. This will reassure your partner—and yourself—that the cycle of resentment and anger can change.

How Understanding Differences Can Lead to Trust

As discussed earlier, we all have both male and female "energy," which is simply a way to describe how men have what are considered female qualities and women have what are perceived as male qualities.

Male energy is very directed. Male energy wants to get to the next destination; it wants to reach the final climax, whether in bed, in an argument, or in a career. Male energy is what gets us to the next level. These traits are a great way to get things done, but they can sometimes be perceived as insensitive to feelings.

Women want men to take charge. This makes women feel safe. This, however, does not mean women want to be controlled.

Feminine energy is "in the moment." Sometimes female energy is experienced as a force that digs in and will not let go. Female energy is in the present and experiences all of the senses. Female energy is the sensual and creative force behind our relationships.

Male energy wants to solve problems; female energy wants to experience the emotions until there is a relief of tension. This can lead to stress between partners, misunderstandings, and anger. If a woman is upset, she will want to talk about it until the energy is spent. If a man is upset, he will devise a way to "fix" the problem. For men, listening to women talk endlessly about their feelings can be frustrating. If a woman continues to talk about the problem after the man has offered his advice, he may become resentful, feeling like she did not appreciate the solution he came up with for her. A woman will experience this as a shutdown of her feelings. She will resent his trying to "fix" her and feel like he is not listening to her when she wants to talk. Understanding these differences can lead to greater trust and less need to act out anger and resentment.

For example, one of the sexiest things a male partner can do is to be directive. Women want men to take charge. This makes women feel safe. This does not mean women want to be controlled, and it is important for anyone in a relationship to feel he or she has a voice. But there is something about a man taking charge in bed that appeals to feminine sexuality. Many couples are intrigued by the capacity to channel their anger and resentment into sexuality in a healthy way.

On the other hand, couples who build resentment between them have a tendency to withdraw from each other, and move farther apart. What if that resentment could be verbalized, perhaps through a healthy dialogue, and then channeled into a strong and passionate sex life? What if, instead of withdrawing into our cave, we could integrate it into our sexual partnerships? What would that look like?

Think about the romantic paperback novels where the man throws the woman on the bed and they make mad, passionate love. There is sometimes a sexiness that comes from having sex that is a little "rougher." Not all women can play this game. They need to feel comfortable and secure before lovemaking, but if they can surrender to the passion and the power, the sex can be even better than "make up" sex. It can be "work through it before the argument" sex!

Surrendering to the Moment— and to Our Partner

The more we trust our partners and let them in, the more confident they will feel. The more we can surrender, or let go, the more our partners can please us. Receiving love in the form of sensual pleasure can be more of a challenge than giving love and sensual pleasure. We need the safety of healthy boundaries to surrender to the moment. If we trust that anger can be managed and worked through, then this will allow us to relax and receive.

One way to redirect the angry energy is to reawaken the inner adult. The inner adult is different from the inner child. We all have an inner child—a youngster that lives in us from our childhood. Don't we all act like six-year-olds in our relationships sometimes?

We tend to behave at our lowest possible functional level at home and with those we love and feel safest with. Remember having a good day at school, and then getting off the bus and acting cranky with Mom? You were tired and stressed, and when you were home with loved ones you could express your frustration. We sometimes act like six-year-olds as adults, too.

Recognize in an argument that you don't want to be six years old. You want to be an adult. You want to recognize that when you feel like your inner six-year-old, it's because something is happening that reminds you of your childhood. Then tell your partner how you feel, using the Imago dialogue. It might sound like:

"When you say that to me it makes me feel X and that reminds me of when I was a kid and Y."

Partners should simply mirror back what you are saying, if they are able to. Or, if they are very angry, ask them whether they can validate your feelings for you.

One way to redirect the angry energy is to reawaken the inner adult.

Invite your adult self to the conflict. How does it want to act? Think about responding intentionally instead of being reactive to what your partner triggers in you.

For example, if we want to be our inner adult in our relationship, we need to communicate as an adult partner. Being direct and honest and not withholding feelings can all lead to a new connection. If you can't resolve all of your issues in one sitting, don't be afraid to go to bed! Your erotic life can help work out your issues for you, just like the couple in the following case.

Working Out Anger in Bed

Average husband closes his book and reaches over to turn off his bedside lamp. Typical wife rolls over away from him in her sleep, pulling all the covers onto her side of the bed. He lies awake on his back, feeling the distance between them. The resentment that has been between them for years has been creating distance and friction in the relationship.

He is afraid that if he wakes her up to have sex, she will be angry and complain about having to get up in the morning. This makes him feel like he is being criticized by one of his parents. He feels a moment of pain and frustration and tenses his body, not sure if he should roll over and give her the cold shoulder or wake her up to argue with her.

Typical wife, half asleep, feels the distance between them. She wonders whether he wants to make love. Part of her wishes he would just try; this would confirm for her that he still finds her attractive even though she has gained weight since the kids were born. She wants him to affirm his love and attraction for her, but she doesn't know how to ask for this. Sometimes she feels abandoned and alone.

Average husband waits and wonders whether she will pursue him. His low self-esteem has been triggered over and over through the lack of sexuality in their relationship. He wonders whether he can really honor his commitment to her and stay married. Why is it called "settling down" anyway? He doesn't feel like he settled for his wife. He knows he was attracted to her for a reason, and wants the relationship to stay erotic and connected.

Typical wife wonders whether her partner still finds her sexually attractive, since he hasn't initiated sex in a while. She used to have such great erotic energy, she thinks. She remembers every fantasy she has ever had, and she wonders about his.

The moment comes when they both take a deep breath, and decide to push their edge, just like in yoga class that morning when the instructor asked them to push through the discomfort of a pose just slightly, finding a new edge, without forcing. She tries to reach out her hand toward him to see if he will respond. He rolls toward her. They both breathe. They lie facing each other, and with eyes open, begin to focus on making eye contact. He reaches out and pulls her closer to him.

"I love you," he says.

"You love me?" she asks.

"Yes, I love you," he says.

"I love you, too," she says, "even though I am so angry at you all the time."

He responds, "So you love me even though you are angry at me all the time?"

"Yes," she says, smiling. They breathe together, slowing down their breath. He begins to stroke her back as he exhales, and she relaxes.

They are on their way to a new connection, and a new erotic and passionate partnership.

The Spiritual and the Physical

Spirituality and sex are intimately and irrevocably linked. Our bodies, minds, and souls unite during sex and connect us to the Divine in a way that no other spiritual work can. Most of the spiritual practices today focus on taking us out of our bodies and away from the physical. Other practices, such as yoga, psychotherapy, and bodywork (in our Westernized versions) eliminate the sexual connection and often skip over the sensual altogether. Incorporating sexuality into a spiritual practice helps us connect to each other and to the spirit of our partners through a deep appreciation of sexuality.

Energy is raised when there is arousal, the observation of time slows down, and sex goes in slow motion. The more aroused we are, the slower and more sensual the dance, and the more spiritually connected we feel.

This next exercise links the spiritual and the sensual so that you and your partner can feel connected on another level. Take your time, enjoy the moment, and appreciate the closeness.

EXERCISE
Spiritual and Sensual Closeness

For this exercise, you will need at least sixty minutes of uninterrupted time. Make sure the children are taken care of, the phone is off, and you have no obligations. Find a quiet, warm space where you and your partner can be together. Lie down facing one another. Find a comfortable position to be as close as possible to each other.

Step One

Breathe deeply into your lower abdomen and exhale longer than you inhale. Try to make your breath an exercise in letting go. Breathe deeply into your pubic area and the root of your spine. Try to match your breath with your partner's. Don't hold your breath. Relax all of your muscles. Gaze into your partner's left eye, the receptive eye. Use your mouth to exhale, making any noises that feel comfortable to express. Continue to breathe until you feel a rise of energy in your genital area.

Step Two

Rock gently back and forth in your pelvis and hips. Move together without penetration, feeling the experience mesh with your breath. See whether you can feel your partner at a different level as you gaze into his or her soul. Get a sense of who he or she is in spirit.

Step Three

Take turns saying something to each other that you would not normally think of. For example, what is it that you truly want from your partner? Perhaps you have never expressed this before. What is it you long for from him or her?

Have your partner mirror back what you ask. Take longer breaths, breathing into your genitals.

Step Four

Rock back and forth from your hips. When you both become aroused, shift into gentle massage. Stroke your partner on the exhalation only. Take turns. Slowly sweep your hands along your partner's back. Stop and inhale. Take your time. You can move to your partner's chest and eventually the genitals. Massage on the exhalation.

(continued)

Step Five

Use penetration to focus on your rhythm and exhale as you penetrate. Tighten and release your perineum muscles, then relax. Keep the gaze on each other's eyes.

If you feel that you are coming close to orgasm, stop and breathe and gaze into your partner's eyes. Focus on your perineum muscles, tightening and releasing.

Encourage your partner to breathe deeply into the abdomen if his or her breath gets shallow or rapid. Help your partner by slowing down your own breath and continuing eye contact. Do this "pause" several times as you come close to orgasm, pulling back and reconnecting with your partner.

Step Six

When and if you are ready to orgasm, see whether you can breathe deeply and push down while you come. Try to relax, breathing deeply, bearing down, and tightening only your perineum area. Relax into the orgasm. Stay in this position as you come down from orgasm, moving as little as possible and continuing to gaze into your partner's left eye.

Continue to breathe together. Keep eye contact, kiss, and stroke as you both come down.

If you want to, you can begin again.

Tolerating Joy

As is often the case, we become comfortable with our habits. The things we do, the words we say, and even the thoughts we entertain and invite into our minds are patterns that get stronger the more we practice them.

We always get more of what we focus on, whether it's positive or negative. For instance, if we are focused on what we don't like in our relationships, then we may notice that those things seem to increase. If we focus on what brings us joy in our relationship, we feel it more often. For some of us, joy can be almost uncomfortable when we have gotten used to being miserable. Sometimes the moments of true joy in our relationships can feel fleeting. Could it be that when we feel joy we push it away?

Joy is a state of mind and a state of spirit. If we are focused on the joy in our partnerships and learn to sit in that feeling for longer periods of time, we find that more joy comes in and stays around.

The journey toward having a more passionate partnership can be a joy-filled journey! Having a more passionate partnership begins by communicating your erotic needs. The increased sexual connection and passion that result can be used as a foundation to work through all issues in the relationship, creating safe mirroring and decreasing fear and anxiety for the future.

Focusing on the joy of the journey, rather than the final destination, means we can be fully present in our relationship.

EXERCISE
Positive Sexy Flooding

For this exercise, you will need uninterrupted quiet time together. Make sure the kids are taken care of. Set up the room with a romantic atmosphere. Turn the lights down low, light candles, and put out fresh flowers or incense.

The first step of the exercise will be writing down a list of all the things you appreciate about your partner sexually. The second part of the exercise will be taking turns flooding each other with these positive sexual statements. Receiving can be harder than giving. Let yourself be filled up when your partner floods you.

Step One

Find a comfortable place to make a list. Write down all of the things you love and appreciate about your partner sexually. This may include a list that describes how your partner makes you feel, how he or she looks, how your partner touches you, and so on. Anything else you appreciate about your partner sexually should go on this list. Use a few words to describe each appreciation.

Step Two

Decide who will be the sender and who will be the receiver. Receivers should sit in a chair in the center of the room. Senders should walk slowly around their partner, list in hand, and read everything they appreciate, whispering loudly enough in their partner's ear to be heard and leaning down to get as close as possible.

Senders should tell their partners specifically how they appreciate the things they do in bed and how they appreciate each part of their body. They should tell them the things they love to do to them and why, all the while whispering and walking around them. Flood them with sexual appreciation.

(continued)

Step Three

The sender's voice can be louder than a whisper now. Senders should notice how the receiver responds. Senders can say the appreciations in their most sexy voice, letting their partners know with their hands that they love to touch them. They should repeat the appreciations that cause the most reaction.

Step Four

Now switch. Senders become receivers and the new senders send over their list of sexual appreciations.

Step Five

When you are both done and feeling flooded with positive appreciation, move directly into lovemaking if you wish. Or you can take a few moments and share one thing you appreciated about this exercise with your partner. Make sure you mirror your appreciations now in this closing piece. You may feel overwhelmed with positive feelings. You may even feel joy. Allow yourself to have this moment of joy. Before you separate and break your connection with your partner by getting up and moving, let yourself experience the joy for a little longer than you can tolerate.

One of the greatest gifts we can bring to our relationship is to acknowledge the moments of joy, focusing on what it feels like to be truly connected and in our Eros energy. Our creative life force makes us feel passion. Passion makes us feel connected. Being connected brings joy.

In this next exercise, be with your partner in a moment of joy. Find the feelings that make you happy, content, and connected. Tolerate the joy for one more moment than you might normally experience. You deserve it, and so does your partner.

Our creative life force makes us feel passion. Passion makes us feel connected. Being connected brings joy.

EXERCISE
Feel the Joy

Find some time where you can focus on your partnership and the passion that you crave. Make sure the kids are taken care of, the phone is turned off, and you have uninterrupted time to be together. Set up the room for romance and passion. Light candles, turn off the lights, spread rose petals on the bed, and use pillows and blankets that feel sensual on your body. Have lubricant and massage oil handy.

Prepare yourself by taking a warm bath or a hot shower. Shave, moisturize, and take the time to get ready for lovemaking with your partner. Put on sexy lingerie or let yourself be comfortably naked. Anticipate the joy of connection with your partner.

Step One

Make love to an orgasm. You might use one or more of the methods discussed in this book. Take your time. Don't rush to the finish line. Appreciate the journey of getting there together. Let yourself experience with all of your senses what it feels like to be in the moment, making love with your partner.

Step Two

After making love and experiencing an orgasm, kiss your partner but do not speak. Lie together and do not move your body. Let yourself feel the energy that has been created by your lovemaking. Feel the stillness in the room and around you. Let yourself feel the air on your skin. Feel the joy that comes with orgasm and pleasure.

Try to remain still, maintaining the connection with your partner. Touch your partner, but let yourself be still. Appreciate the feeling that spreads out from your genitals to the tips of your fingers and toes. Feel the energy circulate throughout your internal system. Feel the joyful energy of touching another person, physically and spiritually. Feel the joy of being totally in your body and yet out of it at the same time. Notice how far your energy radiates around your body.

Step Three

With your eyes closed, visualize the joy-filled energy as it dissipates, floating into the air around you. Let go of the energy; do not try to hold on to it. Feel the power of the journey.

Step Four

When you are completely back to earth, embrace your partner and settle in for sleep or feel the energy created that will allow you both to move back into the world, energized, alive, and living your most passionate partnership!

ACKNOWLEDGMENTS

I would like to thank my children, Tyler and Emma, for their tireless patience and for being such great people. Thanks to my sister Melanie Barnum for her support. And thanks to Will Kiester at Fair Winds Press, for believing in the potential of this book, and to Cara Connors, for gently guiding my thoughts. Thanks to all my Imago teachers, including Harville Hendrix, Jette Simon, and all of my colleagues and friends who have been there for me and encouraged me to write the book.

Special thanks to all of the couples who have come to me for help and taught me so much. You know who you are.

And thanks, Mom, I feel you smiling down on me.

ABOUT THE AUTHOR

Tammy Nelson, MS, ATR, LADC, LPC, is a licensed psychotherapist with 20 years experience working with individuals and couples, and a certified Imago therapist. She is the founder and executive director of the Center for Healing and Recovery in Connecticut, a holistic psychotherapy center providing psychotherapy, massage, acupuncture, yoga, and other classes that support a balanced, holistic lifestyle.

In her private practice she helps couples increase the passion in their relationships by guiding them through empathetic dialogue and intimate forms of communication. She is a licensed professional counselor, a registered art therapist, and a licensed alcohol and drug counselor.

Tammy leads Imago and sexuality workshops for couples, in addition to workshops based on Harville Hendrix's best-selling book, *Getting the Love You Want*, and his theory of Imago therapy. She is the author of *What's Eating You*, a workbook for young people with food issues.